PRAISE FOR MARIA SABANDO AND *LOVING LIFE AT 50+*

I've had the pleasure of working closely with Maria and can't say enough good things about her! She always radiates positivity and joy. She is full of fun ideas—from her recipes to her workout routines, she always keeps it interesting! She has a special way of putting her own spin on everything she does. Through storytelling, her authenticity and sense of humor can bring a smile to anyone's face.

—Jessica Beck, *chief marketing assistant at M. J. Sabando LLC*

I spent a week working side by side with Chef Maria in her kitchen photographing and sampling these tasty recipes for her wonderful new book. Throughout the course of the shoot, her recipes looked so delicious and tempting I had to restrain myself from digging in before capturing the final images.

The salmon chowder, shishito peppers with white sauce, spaghetti squash marinara with shrimp, and pudding trifle are definitely a few of my favorites. I have to say, everything I sampled was delicious, and Maria was kind enough to send me home at the end of each day with plenty of leftovers. I do enjoy cooking and can't wait to add this new book to my stash of recipes. Thank you, Chef Maria!

—Mark Feaster, *professional photographer*

Loving Life at 50+

MARIA SABANDO

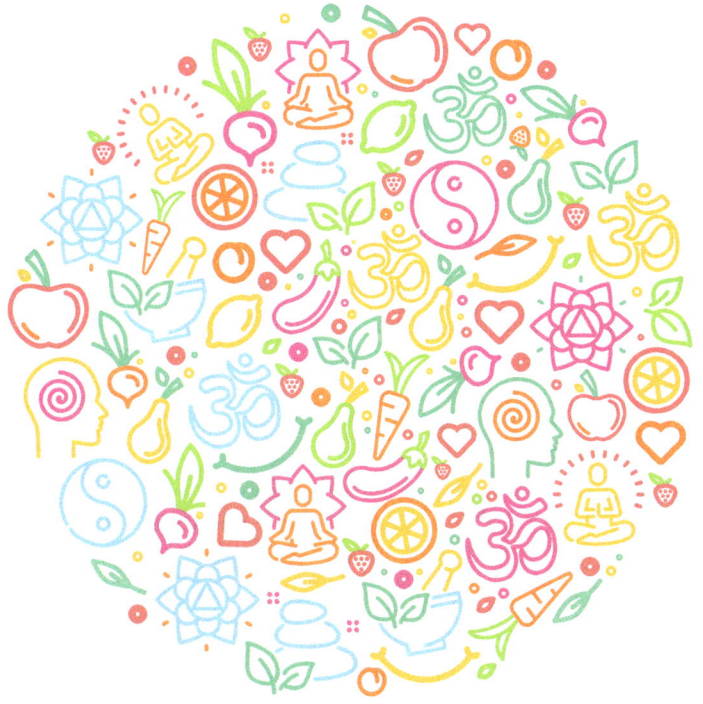

Loving Life at 50+

Embrace Aging through Humor & Wellness

Advantage | Books

Copyright © 2023 by Maria Sabando.

All rights reserved. No part of this book may be used or reproduced in any manner whatsoever without prior written consent of the author, except as provided by the United States of America copyright law.

Published by Advantage, Charleston, South Carolina.
Member of Advantage Media.

ADVANTAGE is a registered trademark, and the Advantage colophon is a trademark of Advantage Media Group, Inc.

Printed in the United States of America.

10 9 8 7 6 5 4 3 2 1

ISBN: 978-1-64225-379-5 (Paperback)
ISBN: 978-1-64225-459-4 (eBook)

LCCN: 2023905823

Cover design by Matthew Morse.
Layout design by Megan Elger.
Photography by Mark Feaster.

This publication is designed to provide accurate and authoritative information in regard to the subject matter covered. It is sold with the understanding that the publisher is not engaged in rendering legal, accounting, or other professional services. If legal advice or other expert assistance is required, the services of a competent professional person should be sought.

> Advantage Media helps busy entrepreneurs, CEOs, and leaders write and publish a book to grow their business and become the authority in their field. Advantage authors comprise an exclusive community of industry professionals, idea-makers, and thought leaders. Do you have a book idea or manuscript for consideration? We would love to hear from you at **AdvantageMedia.com**.

I'd like to dedicate this book to every single member of my family.

However, I want to give special mention to my mother, who, without knowing it, leads by example, with sheer love as her main form of guidance. There is not enough room in these pages to show how she is a trailblazer for those trying to find their way.

My heart is with my beautiful daughters, Alyssa and Emily, without whom there would be no inspiration.

I would also like to thank my sister, Laura, who never hesitates to support me wholeheartedly.

But, most importantly, all my thanks go to my humble, loving husband, Otto, who cannot possibly know how deeply he impacts me with his undying positivity.

Honey, if you were not here, neither would be this book or my "sanity." I am whoever I have become because of you. Thank you to the moon and back.

And to all my lovely friends who stick by me, you know who you are.

Special thanks to all the editors at Advantage | Forbes Books, as well as Mark Feaster, Jessica Stuecher, Lynn Nichols, and all those special friends at NGNG Enterprises. You never plan on meeting angels along the way, but you do!

CONTENTS

INTRODUCTION 1

CHAPTER 1 7
You're over Fifty—Now What?
    Greek Omelet

    Yogurt Parfait

    Eggs Florentine

CHAPTER 2 23
Loving Your Over-Fifty Body
    Blueberry Oatmeal Muffins

    Apple Sandwiches

    Avocado and Hummus Egg

    Yogurt Sundae

CHAPTER 3 47
A Fresh Start
    Pear Brie Salad

    Tuna Pasta Salad

    Salmon Chowder

    Kale Smoothie

CHAPTER 4 63
Lighten Up
    Spicy Cinnamon Popcorn

    Fruit Smoothie

CHAPTER 5 .... **77**

Journal Your Way to Happiness

- Sunday Gravy
- Salad Extraordinaire
- Spaghetti Squash Marinara with Scallops or Shrimp
- Prosciutto Banana Pepper Pizza

CHAPTER 6 .... **95**

Get Inspired!

- Pizza Dulce Cheesecake
- Baked Apple
- Berry Salad
- Banana Bread Pudding

CHAPTER 7 .... **115**

Dining with Others

- Sausage and Arugula Pizza Strips
- Shishito Peppers with White Sauce
- Pesto Shrimp

CHAPTER 8 .... **129**

Keep the Flames Burning

- Gazpacho Shots
- White Sangria Spritzer
- Maria's Bloody Mary
- Twisted Lemon Cocktail

CHAPTER 9 .... **145**

Indulge or You'll Bulge

- Mac 'n' Cheese Supreme
- Eggplant Parmesan
- Air Fryer Chicken Tenders and Fries

CHAPTER 10 163

Dress Your Best

- Pudding Trifle
- Pepper Steak

CHAPTER 11.................181

Party for Health!

- Varied Taco Bar
- Tofu Soup
- Antipasti
- Red Sangria
- Carrot Muffins
- Sherbet Punch

CHAPTER 12 199

Spice It Up, Jazz It Up

- Ecuadorean Ceviche
- Spicy Corkscrew Pasta Salad
- Sausage and Peppers

CHAPTER 13 213

Feast on Life

- Brown Rice Salad
- Skillet Chicken Thighs

ABOUT THE AUTHOR.................225

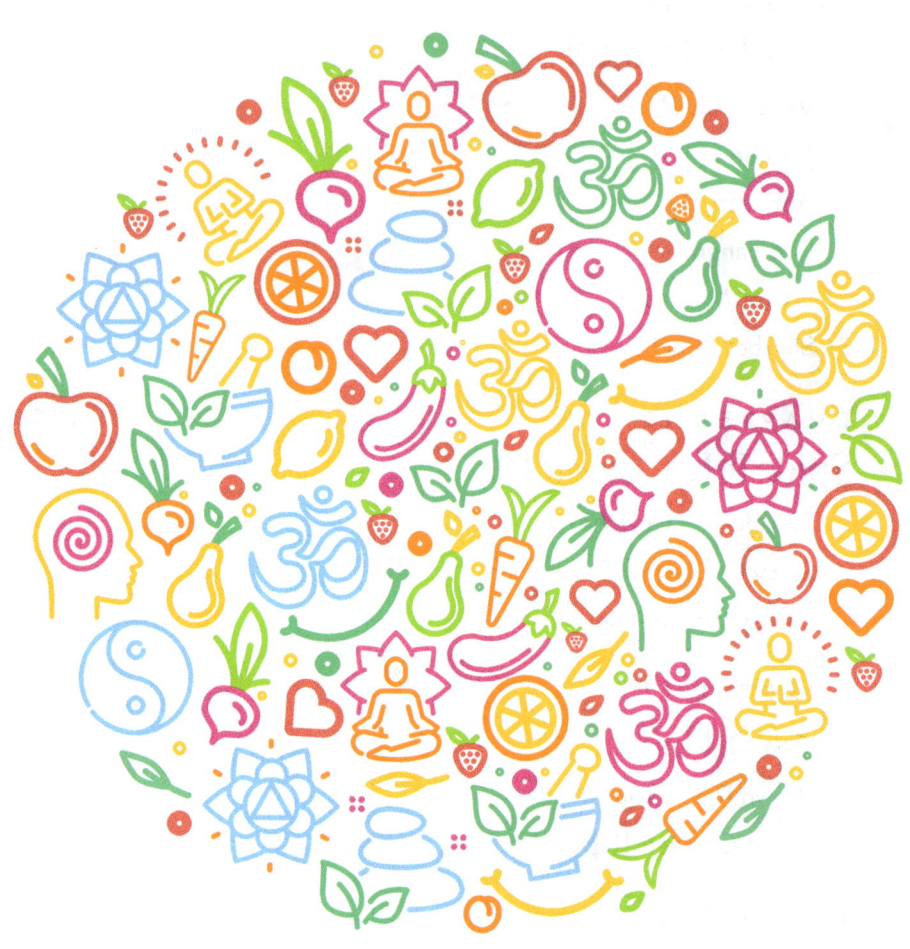

INTRODUCTION

I have a lot of sayings. Some are inspirational; many of them are funny. You'll get a taste of my sayings throughout this book. One of my favorites is "Life is love; love is family; life is family." I express my love for my family in a lot of ways, but a main way is cooking. No surprise I'm Italian! My grandparents emigrated from Sicily to the United States, and they brought with them a legacy of recipes and an appreciation for cooking and all things food. My own love of cooking started as a child, as I watched my mom make homemade marinara, antipasti, and lasagna from scratch. If I were to define Italian cooking, I would say that it is exceptional ingredients assembled with love and inspiration.

Through the years, I've spent hundreds of hours watching cooking shows, and I own more cookbooks than my local library. I've created hundreds of my own recipes, which you will find throughout this book and on my website, officialmariasabando.com. While based in Italian cooking, my recipes incorporate tastes from Asian, American, and French cuisine as well. I'm happy to share my recipes with you.

My favorite part of the day is sitting down to a delicious home-cooked, multicourse family dinner where we pass around dishes and dish about our days. It's what truly fills me up. You'll discover that this book, while being a guide to living your best life in your fifties, is also a little about being a mother, although you don't have to be a mom to enjoy it. There's real truth to the saying "If Mom's not happy, no one is happy."

I know it's accurate in my own home, where my mood spreads faster than wildfire! I'm a proud mother of two beautiful, smart, kind young women, Elissa and Emily. They keep me young, and they keep me laughing. It's female power all around, except for my husband, Otto, who is a doctor and who helped guide this book. My love of food, while mostly wonderful, has had its downsides. I have struggled with weight my entire life, even from a very young age. Name any fad diet, and I've probably tried it, or a version of it. When the diet worked, I'd ride high on the roller coaster of emotions, feeling gleeful that my body was cooperating and I was looking more like the image in my head that I

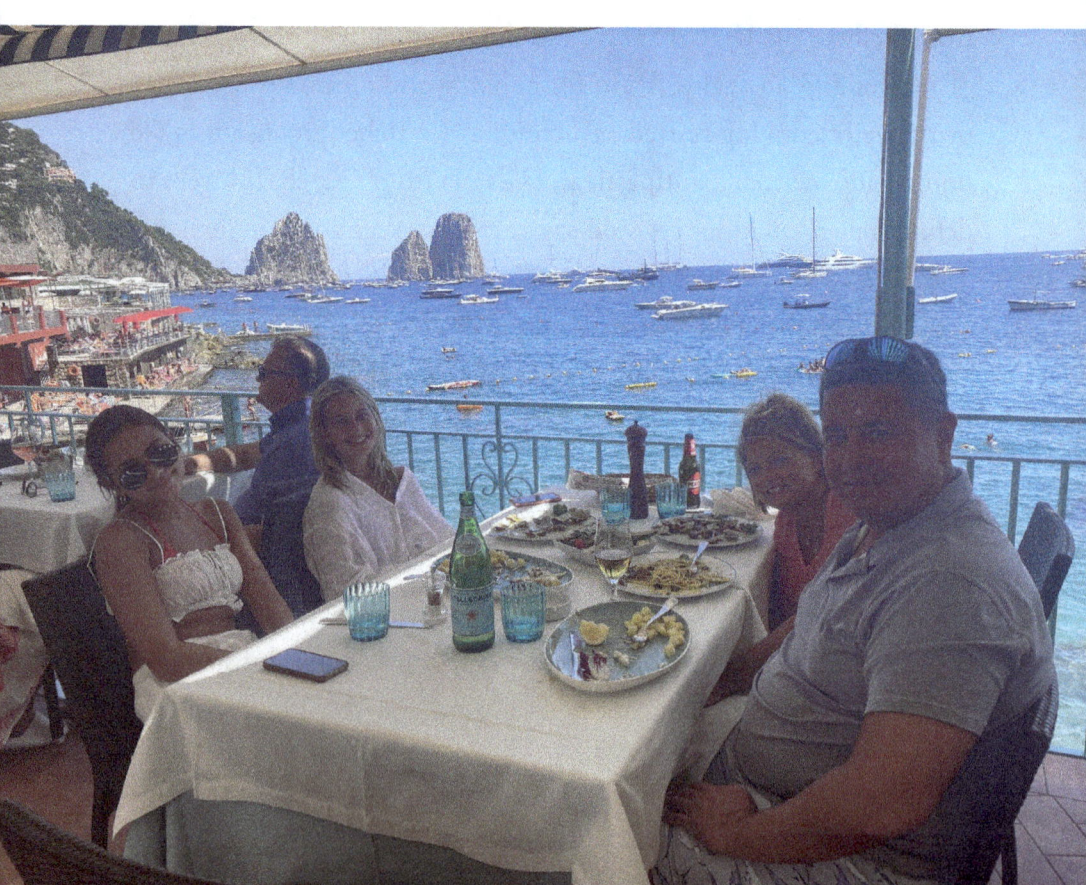

thought I needed to achieve. Other times I worked very industriously at sticking to the diet, but the scale wouldn't tip in my favor.

Like many teenagers in the mid-'80s, I had an unrealistic idea of what a woman should look like, and it seemed there was only one option—beautiful, tall, and exceptionally thin. (Thanks, *Charlie's Angels* and *Vogue*!) The trouble is that I'm short, and every calorie beelines to my hips. So in college I was determined to ace more than my classes. I was obsessed with exercising and controlling my eating, and I became painfully thin. I was hungry all the time, and that's the way I thought it should be. Hunger led to being thin, and being thin meant being happy.

Besides instilling a love of food in us, my Italian grandparents also instilled the idea that thin was better and that you should watch your breadsticks. One of my grandfather's favorite sayings was "Some people live to eat. I eat to work." His message would always get a chuckle, but as a teenager I registered an underlying meaning: you shouldn't make food the center of your life. On its face, it's not a bad message, but when I'd get stuck in the dreaded cycle of bingeing and restricting food that comes with constant dieting, it would elicit some guilt and bad feelings.

Then a beautiful thing happened. One day in my forties, I looked in the mirror and I stopped and asked myself, "Who am I doing this for?" The answer was "Other people."

I decided right then and there that the only person I needed to please was myself. That didn't mean I wanted to let everything go, but it meant that I could loosen up and readjust the standards I was living by. I could eat balanced, nutritious, yet tasty meals instead of starving myself. I could exercise for muscle tone and fitness without killing myself. I could look amazing—and *feel* amazing—without aiming to be ultrathin.

As the years of my youth, my young motherhood, and my early middle age accumulated and swept by, I redefined that made-up image of what I should look like, and I figured out a recipe for my life, one where I maintain my weight while still enjoying delicious food. One where exercise isn't a chore that I have to endure but rather something that energizes me and brings me peace. Most of all, my life recipe empowers me to love myself just the way I am and frees me to grab life by the horns, hold on tight, and enjoy the ride.

If you are reading this book, there's a good chance you are approaching fifty yourself or you've already crossed the line. Well, congratulations! You've made it into middle age. You are wise and wonderful, and you know a thing or two about living. Let's celebrate that and find humor in it together! And if you haven't turned fifty yet, this book will help you cross that line when the time comes. Every day is a gift, and if today is not a good day, know that your next great day is right around the corner. Watch out, world, we fifty-plus women are redefining ourselves, and we know a thing or two!

I hope you are inspired by my personal journey of learning to feel fabulous in my fifties. In the coming pages, I share stories from my life and offer insights on turning fifty, along with a lot of tips and tricks on maintaining a healthy weight and a healthy attitude, including ideas on how to eat to look your best (don't worry, starvation isn't one of them)! Best of all, I encourage you to laugh with me along the way.

In each chapter, watch for

- a selection of inspired, simple recipes that you likely have the ingredients in your kitchen to try right now;
- a new yoga pose at the end of each chapter (I invite you to enter a calm space and leave your worries behind by giving yoga a try—consider it a gift to both your body and your mind);

- interesting health tidbits and fresh ideas sprinkled (like salt) and spilled (like good wine) throughout the book; and

- my famous sayings, which will hopefully inspire you to make a healthy shift or provide a healthy dash of humor to make you smile.

Don't worry, I won't leave you hanging when you high-five me for helping you find an activity that's your passion, plan a fun party, or discover new ways to keep the flames of your relationship burning (or when I suggest ways to manage other burns that are much less desirable, like the hot flashes that come with menopause). I'll even help you find the perfect outfit right in your own closet!

Come along and explore with me a new way to be at fifty-plus. We've got a lot to cover, so let's get started!

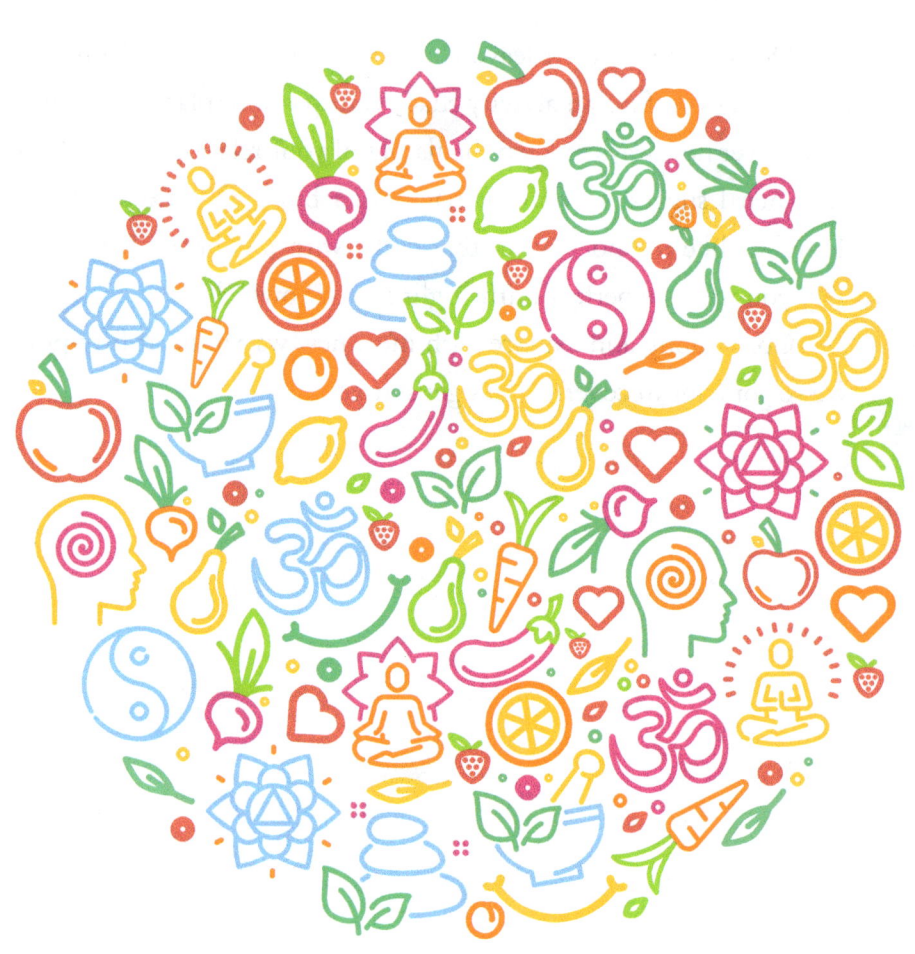

CHAPTER 1

You're over Fifty—Now What?
Reset with Eggs Florentine

It happened when I was in my midforties, probably about the same time it happened to you.

It's something that happens to all of us maturing women.

I had just worked out at the gym, and I was feeling especially energized and young. I swung by the grocery store to do some weekly shopping, and I was minding my own business in the checkout lane. It was busy, the line was long, and my cart was full. When I finally reached the register, I was putting in my bank card to pay when I heard someone offering to help some old lady with her groceries.

But the old lady wasn't answering, and I heard him say it again: "Ma'am? Ma'am? Do you need some help unloading the items from the bottom of your cart?"

What? Wait a minute. I whipped my head around and looked at him. Was he talking to me? There was no way he was talking to me! But he was. I couldn't believe it. Me, a ma'am? Yep. I had just been called "ma'am" for the first time, and it was devastating. Naturally, I turned down his offer to help!

Since that day, I've talked to many friends about their own first "ma'am" experience. If you ask a woman in her fifties if she remembers that moment, you will likely hear a similar story in stark, scorn-filled detail (unless, of course, she's from the South, where women hear "ma'am" from a young age). For many of us, it's a weird coming-of-middle-age moment that draws an imaginary line in the sand. On one side is youth; on the other, old age. Maybe for the first time we realize that the world is seeing us as older women, and it starts our wheels turning. We wonder, Is that what I really am? An older woman?

After the initial shock of hearing "ma'am" for the first time wore off, I started thinking about that imaginary line, and the more I thought about it, the more I decided it was bunk. Why can't I have one foot in my youth and let it ground me as I step into my later years? Even if the mirror doesn't reflect my younger self, my spirit does, and that's what really counts. The label that strangers give me doesn't matter. I get to choose, and I choose my youthful self. If someone wants to assume I'm old, let 'em. One of the perks of growing older is that you stop caring so much what other people think. It's liberating. And sometimes it's downright funny.

The other morning, we were enjoying a lovely family breakfast. I had just made a batch of my delicious Greek Omelets. We were discussing family vacations, and I was telling my daughters, Emily and Elissa, about going to the Bahamas as a teenager, and my youngest daughter, Emily, asked, "Did they have planes back then?"

I mean, sometimes all you can do is laugh.

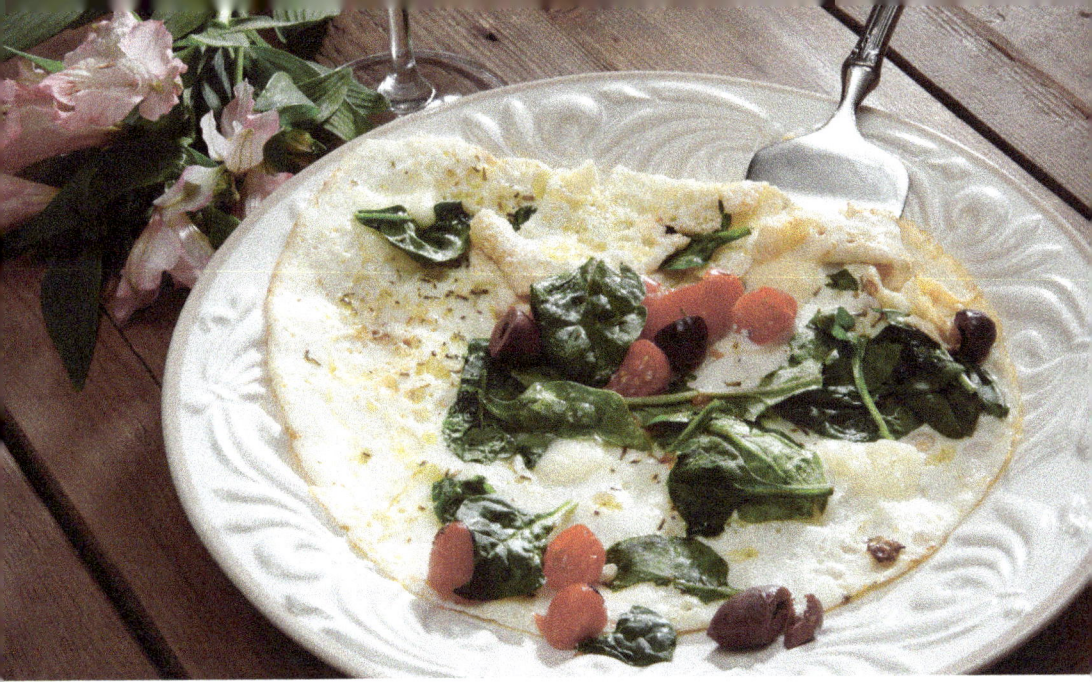

Greek Omelet

- 3 tablespoons olive oil
- ⅓ cup egg whites
- ½ teaspoon salt
- ½ teaspoon rosemary
- ½ cup fresh baby spinach
- ½ cup feta cheese
- Brine or water
- ¼ cup calamata olives
- ½ cup tomato

Chop the olives and tomatoes, and cut cheese into 1-inch cubes. Warm the frying pan over medium heat. Add oil and twirl around in the pan. Add egg whites and cook 2 minutes. Add salt, rosemary, spinach, feta cheese, olives, and tomatoes. Cook 3 to 5 more minutes. Serve open faced or fold in half.

I revel in hanging out with my daughters and absorbing their youthful energy. Some people say teenagers are hard to raise, but I see them as a blessing. They help keep me young. I know I can't go back in time and be a teenager or young woman again, but hey, I can still rock it like a teenager. Especially where it counts—the gleeful, silly joy that bubbles up and releases like a delicious glass of bubbly.

I understand that aging is hard. Especially in a society that values youth and beauty. When you turn fifty, you are not quite an old lady, but you are not a spring chicken either. People don't know how to deal with that. Should they call you ma'am or miss? Should they offer to carry your groceries or not? It's up to each of us to tell them how to treat us. What age do you want to be? I say you decide, because holding on to the strength and bravado from when you were a young woman is half the battle.

Numbers on the scale, or numbers of years, are just numbers. Maybe you get upset about the number, but no one else cares. Why torture yourself? The number means literally nothing. You can look and feel great. Ask yourself, Is it time to stop trying to live up to an old expectation of an ideal weight? Notice that little voice that's telling you what you should and shouldn't look like. If it's based in old messages, shift it. Each time you hear it, choose to focus on what brings you happiness instead. Over time, you will change your expectations and feel the freedom in doing so.

You can be a young old person or an old young person; it's your choice.

Fifty is the new [insert any age here]. Don't act your biological age; act your spiritual age. Do you feel like a teenager that's peering out from behind your mature eyes (and yeah, maybe sometimes when you catch your reflection in the mirror you think, Who is *that*)?! Regardless, that's great news! Because how you feel on the inside is what matters most. Maybe you feel your real age but you are lucky enough to have a body that's free of aches and pains. More power to you! Or maybe you feel the aches and pains but you decide you are going to power through them and do what you want, regardless. Even better yet.

The point is you can have a young mentality even when you are old. Maybe you can't stay out all night like you could when you were young, and likely you no longer want to, but you can still have new experiences. No matter your age, you can create a bucket list and envision completing it (see mine in chapter 6). As of this writing, I'm fifty-three. I've never been to the Grand Canyon, but I'm determined to check it off my list. It might be a modified version (i.e., hiking into the canyon but riding a mule out), but I can still get it done. Bucket list items don't have to be as big—literally—as the Grand Canyon. Maybe your bucket list involves a weekly date between you, a great cup of coffee, and a bookstore. Or you, a friend, and an overnight shopping trip in the city. The beautiful thing is that you get to decide. Trying new things feeds your younger spirit and keeps you young where it counts the most—on the inside.

> **The strength that you had when you were young is still in you. You can feel excited about experiencing new things and awe when you make them happen. It's all attitude, and it's all you.**

Don't forget that the older you in the mirror is also the wiser you and the more liberated you. A real benefit to aging is that you stop caring so much what people think. You've lived this long, and you've come this far. You know things. Long ago, you figured out how the world works, how to maintain relationships, and the value of money. You know that what matters the most in life is not turning heads (or matching some ideal in your own head) or how much money you have; it's knowing yourself and accepting who you are and respecting all of the experiences over the years that brought you to where you are today. Let wisdom be your guide.

You are aging, and that's okay. You no longer have to wear giant hoop earrings and skinny jeans (unless you want to)! Nor do you have to dress like an old woman. I have memories of family gatherings when my huge Italian family would come together for dinner, and it was always the same—the men were in the living room discussing business, and the women were in the kitchen preparing the food, wearing those awful matronly black dresses. Being stuck in old stereotypes is just that—old thinking. Today, there's new thinking, and we as powerful women in our fifties get to lead the way in defying stereotypes and resetting the idea of what an older woman should look like, act like, and feel like. It's about time!

Let's hit the reset button on a few things. For starters, weight isn't just a number on the bathroom scale. It's how we move and how we feel inside our bodies. It's the way we present ourselves and how we choose clothing that flatters us. We get to decide what we want to look like and what our look will be. Choose to look and feel fabulous.

In the upcoming pages, I share insights on how I moved beyond the scale and adopted a broader, more spacious view of health and wellness. In this new expanse, I've had the room to really explore my relationship with food and come up with meals that work for me—food that fills me up but doesn't overstuff, such as balancing pasta with vegetables. I've got hundreds of recipes (sign up on my website, officialmariasabando.com), and every day another one percolates to the surface. They are all tasty, and they are nearly all healthy, with a little room for dessert. The days of starvation and yo-yo diets are officially over! I say indulge or you bulge. (It's one of my playful mantras you'll learn about later in the book.)

A healthy body is about so much more than maintaining a certain weight. Of course, maintaining your weight so that you feel good about yourself is important, but having a healthy body, one you feed with nutritious foods that give you energy to do the activities that you love to do, like yoga or spending time with family and friends, is what truly makes you feel young. Being fit, feeling toned, and experiencing the energy that comes from living a healthy life is much more important than achieving a set number on the scale. It is your ticket to happiness.

A part of feeling good is finding peace with yourself when you look in the mirror, and that's a very personal relationship each woman has with herself. I've created guidelines around eating that are relaxed but still have bumper lanes. Sticking to these guidelines, like minding portion size, helps me stay consistent with my weight. I'll share these guidelines with you throughout the book, and if they resonate with you or if they spark the creation of your own healthy habits around eating and exercising, I'm truly honored.

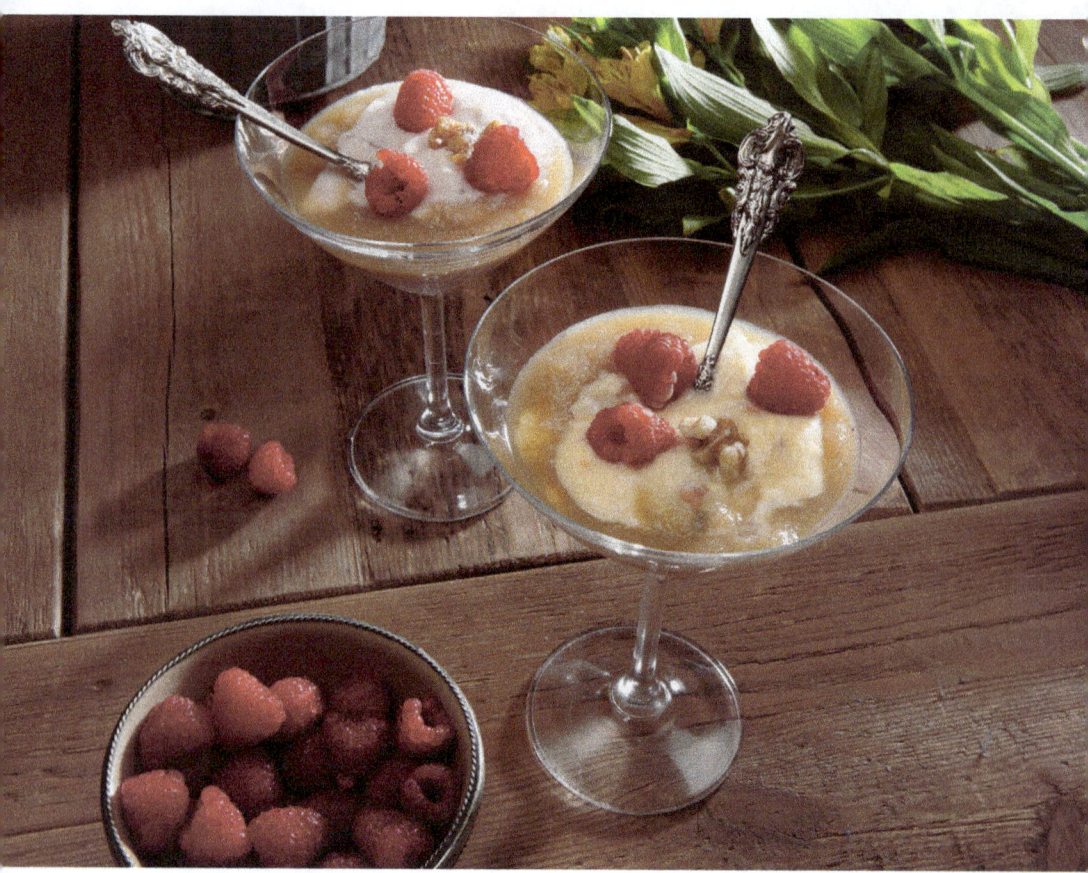

Yogurt Parfait

1 small container Greek yogurt, any flavor (I like peach or berry)

2 tablespoons chopped walnuts

Sprinkle of berries

1 teaspoon cinnamon

¼ cup unsweetened applesauce

Mix yogurt with cinnamon. Layer all ingredients except walnuts in a wine glass. Top with chopped walnuts.

Of course, coming to peace with yourself and finding the right balance that works for you with nutritious eating, exercise, and positive self-talk and acceptance takes trial and error, so I urge you to be gentle with yourself as you move forward into a new way of being in your fifties. Don't expect to always get it right. It will take time for you to figure out what works for you. After all, you have formed your own unique beliefs and habits around eating and exercise over many years. It takes time to break down what doesn't serve you and replace it with what does. Some of what I say may resonate deeply; other times you might wonder, What is this woman talking about? That's the beauty of it. We are all different, and what motivates you might not motivate others. Yet we all likely have one thing in common—a desire to live our best lives in our fifties.

Over the years, I've shifted my mindset and I've come to accept my body just as it is. After all, we come in all different shapes and sizes, and (usually!) I embrace that mine is just right for me. Being comfortable in your body, no matter what your shape, seems to be where it's at, today. I welcome this shift, and as a woman who is fifty-plus, I encourage you to do the same. It may take some reprogramming from the media messages you received while growing up in the '70s or '80s, but it's worth it.

Whenever you can, try to catch yourself in old ways of thinking, like "Being thin is better," or negative self-talk about your body, like "If only I were a size 8 or a 10." Maybe you need to release comments that you heard growing up from your parents, siblings, or friends. The more you are able to become aware of the old thought patterns that pop in without provocation, the more power you have over changing them. They don't serve you anymore—and probably never did. It's kind of exciting because the more you notice them, the more you begin to look at them objectively. You might even discover where they came from, allowing you to release them and experience healing that lasts. We'll explore this more in chapter 5 when we discuss journaling.

In the past, my sole motivation for exercise was to stay thin. It mostly involved trips to the gym to work out, which often truly felt like work. On the weekends, I'd take hikes or go dancing for fun. As I have matured into my fantastic fifty-plus self, I realize that what's important is simply regular movement. I believe that all movement counts as exercise, whether it is dancing in the kitchen while I cook, walking my Yorkie (named Chip), or having friends over for a yoga session or a group walk followed by brunch. I believe that it's better to move about the kitchen cooking a nutritious meal than it is to go on a run and then reward yourself with your favorite fast food. The calories you burn rarely ever equal the reward calories that you eat. In chapter 2 you'll come to understand that exercise, while wonderful for helping you become fit and toned, is not a dieting tool.

MOVE FOR YOUR BRAIN

According to the Centers for Disease Control and Prevention (CDC), moving every day is not just good for our bodies; it's also good for our brains.[1] The CDC says regular, active movement reduces anxiety, lowers the chance of dementia in older adults, and even boosts executive functioning skills that help us organize, plan, and control our emotions and behaviors. Now that's something to think about!

Besides introducing you to a ton of tasty and nutritious recipes (yes, the two can certainly go together!), I'll also give you a quick course in beginning yoga. For the past decade, it has been my passion sport—my personal reset button that just happens to count as exercise.

---

1 Centers for Disease Control and Prevention, *Physical Activity Guidelines for Americans,* 2nd ed., accessed February 22, 2022, https://health.gov/sites/default/files/2019-09/Physical_Activity_Guidelines_2nd_edition.pdf#page=39.

Maybe you will also develop a love for yoga, but if not, you might take a few helpful tips from it—like deep breathing to calm yourself when you feel anxious or stretches to relieve stiff and sore muscles. In case yoga isn't your thing, I help you explore your own passions when it comes to movement. By doing so, you'll tap into the pleasure of experiencing an internal glow and confidence boost after a fulfilling workout. You'll discover a deep knowing that your favorite movement is not only good for your body but good for your soul.

Now, close your eyes and envision a big, black reset button. Got it? Good. Reach down and push it. Push it hard. From this day on, it's a fresh start. It's a big step into becoming an older yet fantastic woman. I have no doubt that you are already great. But like most aging women, you might need a tweak here or there to make the shift from old habits and beliefs that don't serve you anymore. Come along on a journey to an improved version of yourself, and become a woman who relaxes into life and finds a way of being in the world that's just right for her. It's a shift that redefines what it means to age. A shift that will move you forward with zest and confidence. Welcome to your fresh start!

To celebrate a fresh start, let's do breakfast! I welcome you to try my Eggs Florentine.

Eggs Florentine

- 1 potato, boiled and cut into cubes
- 1 egg
- ½ teaspoon salt
- ½ teaspoon pepper
- ½ cup fresh spinach leaves
- ¼ cup cheddar or Colby Jack cheese cubes
- 1 teaspoon favorite steak sauce
- 2 tablespoons olive oil

Sauté potato cubes in 1 tablespoon oil. Add salt and pepper, and stir-fry until browned. Set aside. Place spinach leaves in the pan with the remaining oil. Crack egg over spinach, allowing it to fry for 2 minutes. Add cheese cubes, allowing them to melt. Plate potato, then spinach with egg mixture, and drizzle steak sauce over the top.

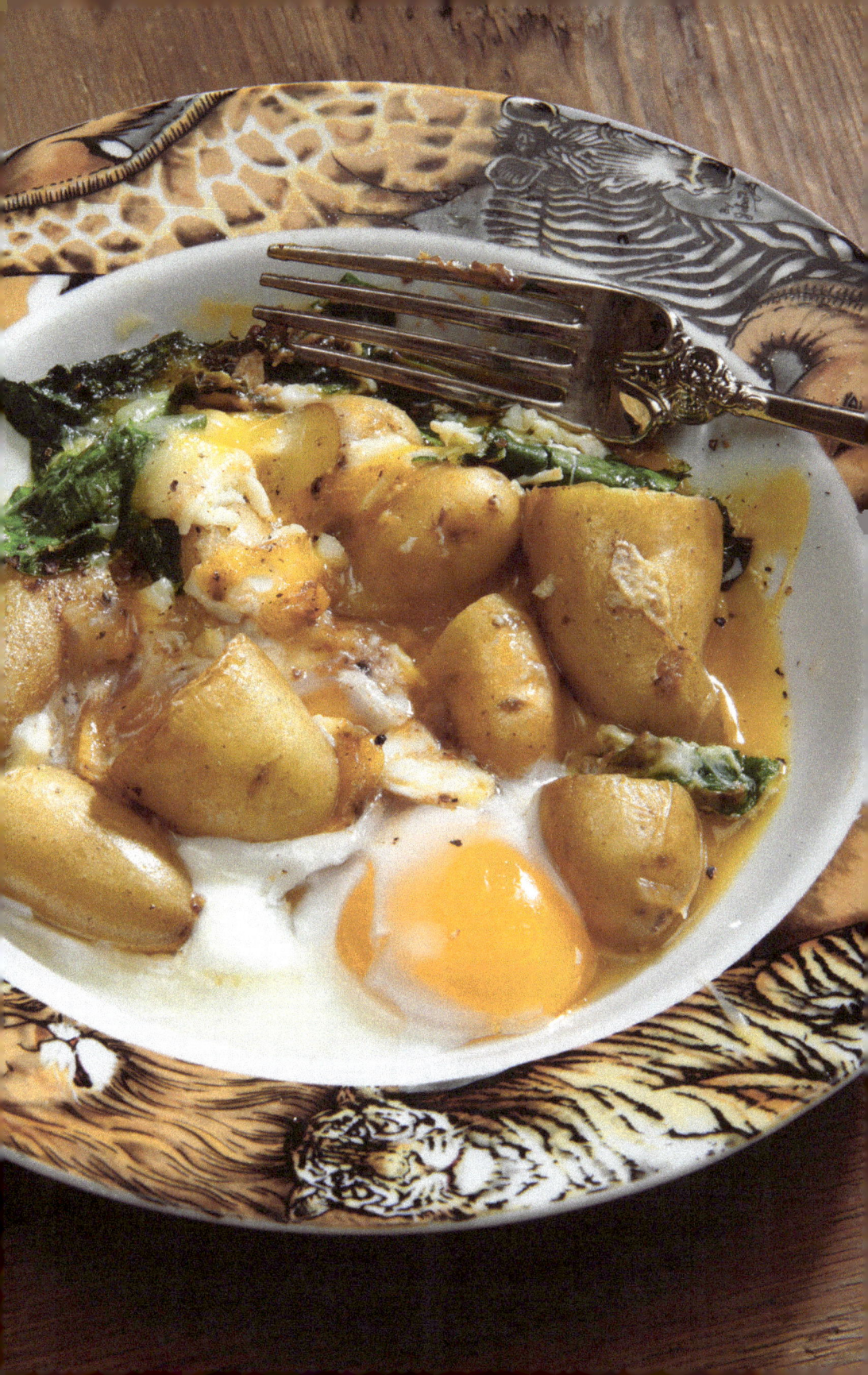

LOVING LIFE AT 50+

CHILD'S POSE

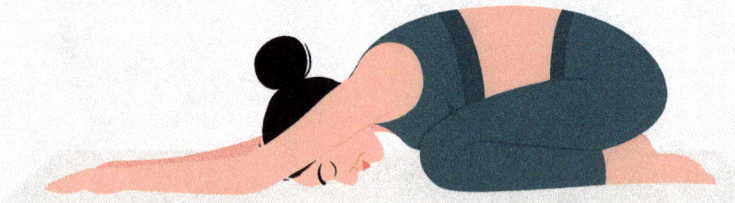

MOVE WITH MEANING

Child's pose is one of the most basic of yoga poses. It's a resting pose that's often done between more challenging positions. Think of it as the reset button of yoga. It's also a great way to start a yoga session, allowing a refreshing stretch of your spine, neck, thighs, and arms. To mark the occasion of embracing a new way of being in your fifties, take a few minutes to give child's pose a try. It feels like giving yourself a hug.

1. Start by sitting on your haunches. Spread your knees wide and bend down, letting your belly rest between your thighs. Resting your forehead on your mat, stretch your arms out in front of you. Inhale deeply. Feel your spine lengthen and your back expand. As you exhale, allow your torso to relax more deeply into the floor.

2. Spend five minutes in child's pose meditating on what it means to you to be a woman who is in, or approaching, her fifties. Breathe deeply. When self-judgment arises, release the negative words in your head with your exhaled breath. Let your mind explore your ideal fiftysomething self. What does she want for her body? For her mind? What brings her joy and meaning? Let ideas bubble up without judgment. If judgment comes, gently counter it with positive affirmations that resonate with you, like "I am beautiful. I am wise. I am strong. My younger self resides within me. Years do not define me. I do."

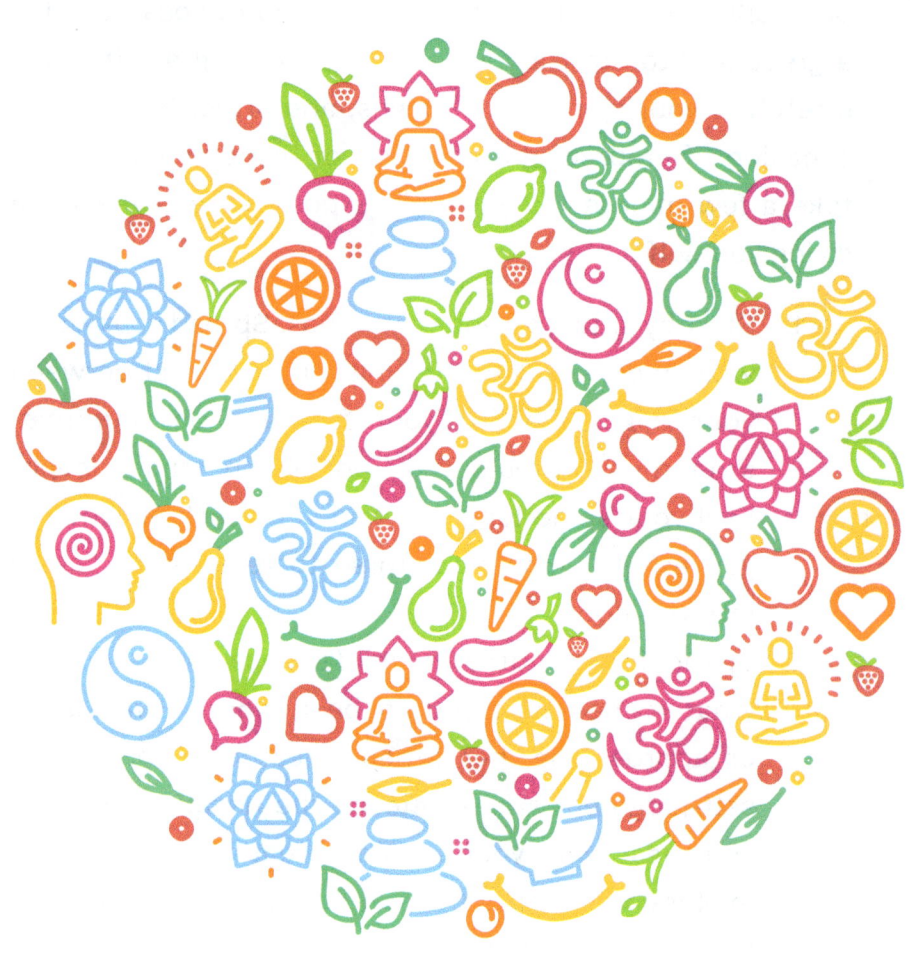

CHAPTER 2

Loving Your Over-Fifty Body
Have Some Fun with Apple Sandwiches

The other morning I woke up feeling groggy because I didn't sleep well, thanks to one too many night sweats. Maybe you can relate. I was moving slow, so I poured myself a second cup of coffee and helped myself to a mid-morning snack of a blueberry oatmeal muffin. Normally, I would be stretching on my yoga mat right about now, or taking Chip, my Yorkie, for a walk.

Blueberry Oatmeal Muffins

¼ cup maple syrup

¼ cup unsweetened applesauce

2 eggs, beaten

¼ cup dairy or almond milk

½ teaspoon vanilla

1 cup whole wheat flour

¾ cup oats

¼ teaspoon baking powder

¼ teaspoon salt

½ cup blueberries

⅓ cup chopped walnuts

¼ cup confectioners' sugar

Spray muffin tin with cooking oil. Mix syrup, applesauce, eggs, almond milk, and vanilla in a large bowl. In separate bowl, combine flour, oats, baking powder, and salt. Add dry mixture to wet and mix well. Add blueberries and stir lightly. Spray muffin cups with oil, then fill with ½ cup batter per cup. Sprinkle nuts over each muffin. Bake at 350°F for 20 minutes. Cool for 10 minutes. Remove from tin with a plastic fork and sprinkle with confectioners' sugar. Makes 12 muffins.

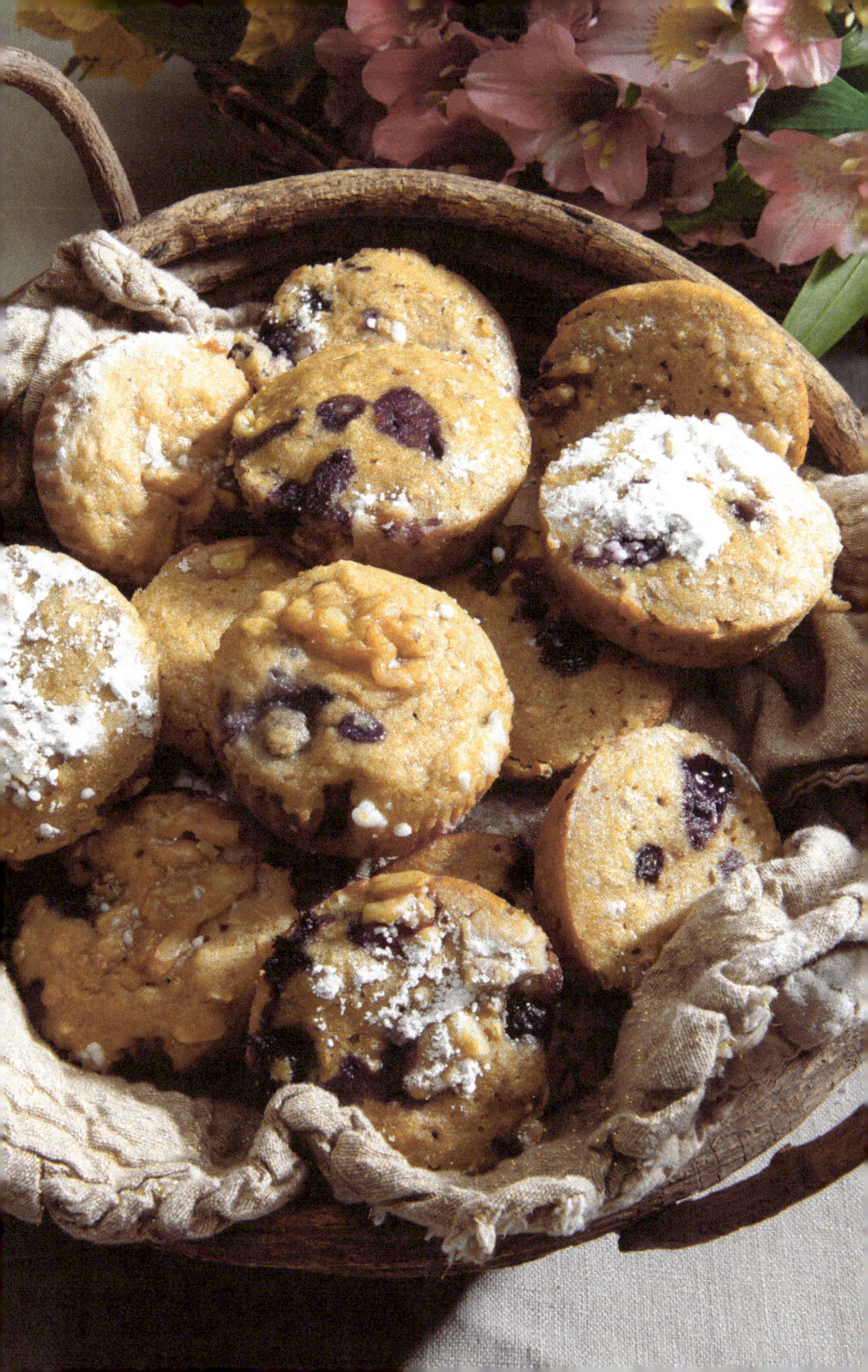

I had just sat down with some bills that needed paying when I heard Emily and Elissa, my teenage daughters, galloping down the stairs like a couple of colts. They sounded insanely perky through my filter of fatigue. When they rounded the corner, they looked even perkier. They were both rocking Lululemon leggings and cropped workout tops. They were laughing and bouncing around the kitchen, filling up their thermal water bottles for spin class. I'll admit. From where I sat with just a sip of liquid energy left in my cup and a pile of bills in front of me, I was feeling a wee bit nostalgic for my own youth. I mean, I am a mother, but I also like to think that I'm a diva!

As the flurry of teenage energy left my house and silence took its place, I found myself chuckling at the irony of it all. I could only shake my head and smile at the contrast between where I'm at in life and where my girls are. Yes, I may be older, and I may never fit into those size 0 stylish leggings ever again, but I can wear a size 8 in a different brand and look—and more importantly feel—pretty darn good. I'm done trying to squeeze myself into something that doesn't fit and that's not comfortable. That goes for both clothing and everything else, from my own self-judgment to others' expectations. Most importantly, nothing fills me up more than the satisfaction of being a mom and watching my daughters revel in their youth, full of energy and hope for what lies ahead.

Sitting there, I also acknowledged the flip side to the joy of having children. If you've raised teenagers, you have likely weathered some stormy seas. All that blaring sun, wind, and rain, and the occasional tornado, has made you tough.

Have you noticed how things in the past that might have bothered you, like an insensitive comment from an acquaintance, don't bother you so much anymore? Today when someone teases me, I usually just laugh rather than second-guess their meaning. We are imperfect beings after all, and that's just how it is. If we were all perfect, we'd all be the same, and what a boring world that would be! If we try to be good at something that doesn't fit with our nature, it often backfires, and we feel bad about ourselves. (That's not to say you shouldn't try new things—just honor who you are.)

I should be this. I should be that. Well, I'm done with that too. We should ban the word "should" from our vocabulary! Maybe you already have, and if so, I applaud you. It's part of our wisdom as older, middle-aged women. We earned this age, so let's celebrate it. We own what we are good at and we let go of the rest.

However, I do enjoy letting imperfection challenge me. I always loved writing growing up; I was even the editor of my middle school newspaper. But somewhere along the way, I got the message that I wasn't a great writer, so I shrunk back in high school. I got an inferiority complex about it—which added fuel to an unhealthy relationship with food in college. Today, I'm able to look at it for what it is. While I'm sad for that dejected young woman, I'm glad I was able to take the challenge and start writing again.

It's like my friend's T-shirt says: "Don't mess with me, I have three daughters." That kind of tenacity makes it easier to love myself and my body a little more with each year that passes. My body is like an old warship that demands respect. It's what allowed me to push the bills aside, honor my current speed, and go do some long, slow stretches on my yoga mat in the morning after my girls left. Taking action that honors myself leaves me feeling centered and satisfied.

By now, you get that yoga is my exercise of choice. I understand it might not be yours. I want you to think of yoga as a metaphor for exercise. What's your yoga? You likely have a good idea of what you enjoy, but if you need a little help, think back to what you enjoyed doing as a kid. When we find ways to exercise that feel like fun, we tend to integrate them into our daily lives. Maybe you were a roller queen who loved to skate around the rink in junior high. Or maybe you loved hitting the tennis ball around the court, like I did, or riding your bike fast down the hills in your neighborhood.

Whatever it was that brought you joy, bring it back into your life today. If you have Rollerblades from the '90s, pull them out and swap out the old wheels for some fresh ones and take yourself to a bike path. If tennis feels like too much to tackle, try pickleball at your gym or through a class offered by your city's recreation department. How about tapping into the freedom that only riding a bike can bring and take a few loops around the neighborhood or take a ride to a nearby park? Once you find your yoga, it will be an anchor for you both physically and emotionally.

After you do an activity, take a break to have a morning or afternoon snack. We are all different, but sticking to an eating pattern of breakfast, morning snack, lunch, afternoon snack, and dinner works great for me for maintaining a healthy weight. You'll notice that the recipes in this book follow that meal/snack pattern for chapters 1 to 5: breakfast, snack, lunch, snack, dinner. Then I branch off from the daily mundane and have some fun with desserts, mocktails/cocktails, romantic meals, family dinners, girlfriend parties, and more. After all, life is for living!

I don't know about you, but I find snack time to be an almost heavenly experience. Snacks have gotten a bad rap as a source of added calories, but for me having a snack is akin to grazing. It's like a bonus minimeal, which helps keep my blood sugar levels and moods nice and steady throughout the day. If I skip my morning or afternoon snack, I get dizzy, and I can't function. Or I am so starved that I overeat at the upcoming meal. Why do that to ourselves? An Apple Sandwich is one of my favorite morning snacks. Maybe it will become one of yours!

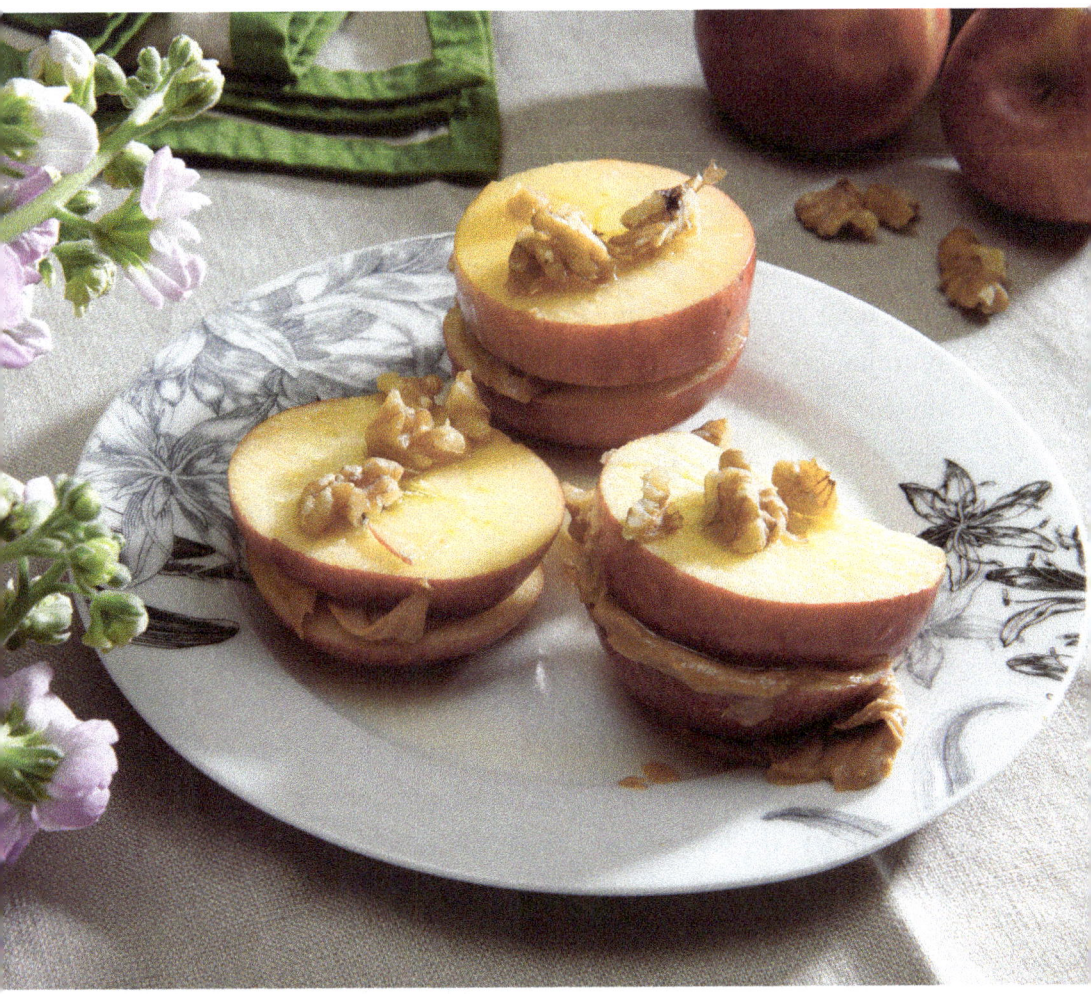

Apple Sandwiches

- 1 apple, sliced into rings
- 1 teaspoon honey
- ¼ cup chopped walnuts
- 1 teaspoon peanut butter

Spread peanut butter on one apple ring. Top with another ring. Drizzle honey on top and add walnuts.

I have a lot of fun mantras that I live by. You probably do, too, because you've lived a while and you know yourself. You know what works for you. One of mine is "Move every day." It's a super easy reminder that I need to get up and move between the time I wake up and the time I go to bed. That's it. No expectations needed. Expectations can take the fun out of movement and make it more like dreaded exercise. Also, listen to your body and honor your headspace. For example, the morning I was tiredly watching my girls literally bound out the door on their way to spin class, I didn't shame myself for not having the energy to join them. Instead, I acknowledged where I was at (tired, sluggish), and I picked a movement to match (stretching and a few simple yoga poses). The opposite is true when I wake up feeling like spring has sprung and I need to spring with it. That's when I do a challenging yoga workout or take a brisk, long walk.

Whether it's 10 minutes of stretching on the floor or a strenuous walk, give yourself a pat on the back and say, "Good job!" no matter how much you moved that day. It all adds up, and it's all good. According to the Centers for Disease Control and Prevention, adults need 150 minutes of moderate-intensity movement each week, along with two sessions of a muscle-strengthening activity each week.[2] The great news is that the 150 minutes can be broken up into convenient chunks. You could commit to 30 minutes of brisk walking (or bike riding, hiking, tennis, swimming, or dancing) each day for five days a week, or you could exchange that for one vigorous aerobic exercise, like jogging, cross-country skiing, spin class, fitness class, etc. for 75 minutes a week instead.

Also, sneak in a little movement whenever you can. Here's a silly idea: While you are heating up your lunch in the microwave at work,

---

2   Centers for Disease Control and Prevention, "Physical Activity Basics," accessed April 4, 2022, https://www.cdc.gov/physicalactivity/basics/adults/index.htm.

do jumping jacks. Or if you have to go down the hall to talk with a coworker, do some speed walking. Heck, it will also help you practice the newfound freedom that aging brings, which is to not care what other people think!

For muscle strengthening, you might need to go to the gym to work your major muscle groups or create a gym at home with hand weights and do good old-fashioned exercises like push-ups, sit-ups, leg lifts, squats, lunges, and strenuous yoga poses like warrior pose or side planks. If this all sounds intimidating, start small and work your way up to these recommendations. And don't forget—gardening, yard work (such as raking and mowing the lawn), and house cleaning all count as movement and exercise! After all this movement, treat yourself to a healthy snack with protein to replenish your muscles, like my Avocado and Hummus Egg.

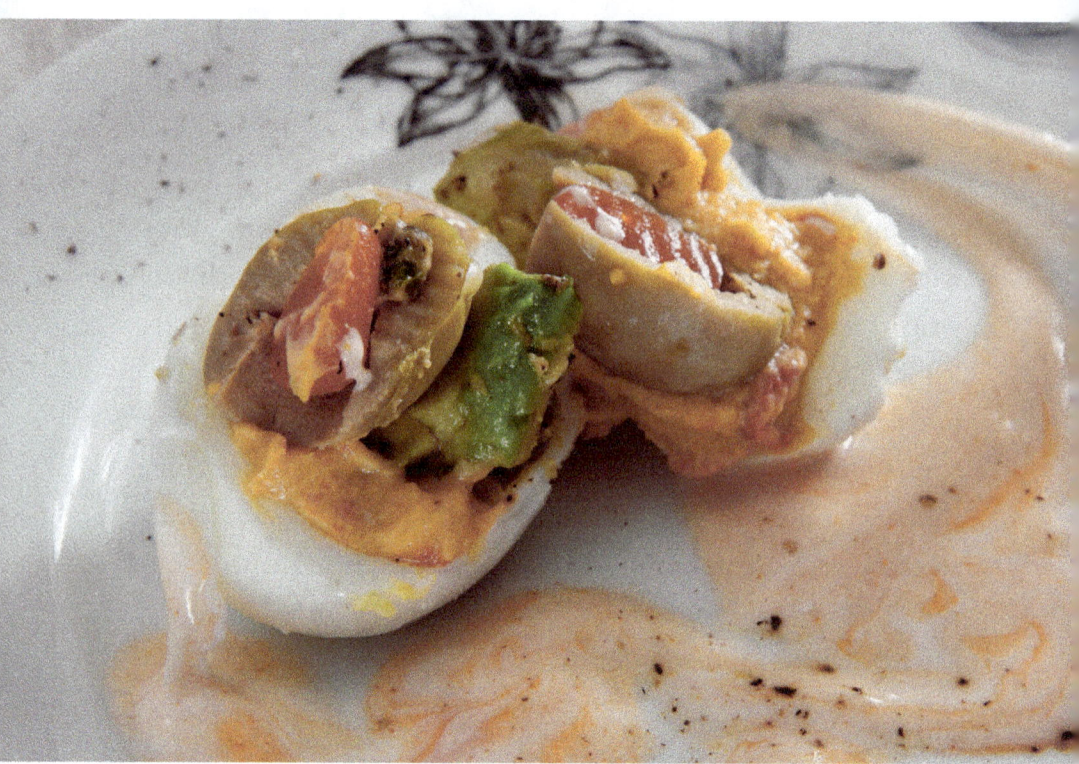

Avocado and Hummus Egg

1 hard-boiled egg, sliced lengthwise
½ ripe avocado, pit removed, and sliced into strips
1 pimento Spanish olive
2 teaspoons hummus

Fill each egg half with avocado and hummus. Top with ½ olive slice for each egg half.

For more tasty and healthy recipes, check out my website at officialmariasabando.com or follow me on Instagram @mariacsabando.

Have you ever noticed that if you get out and move, especially if you are outdoors, you always feel better afterward? That's because our bodies like to move. We are built for it. It's the same with breathing. Breathing is about as natural a movement as you can get, and all movement requires breathing. Studies show that taking deep breaths calms the nervous system. I think it's another reason why I feel so good after yoga. When I start a session, I always begin with some deep breathing to center myself. It shifts my mentality away from whatever I was just preoccupied with to the present. Soon, all I am thinking about is the pose, the stretch, and my breathing. I'm Catholic, and sometimes I wonder if loving yoga and meditation so much is blasphemous. Then I think, "It's so affirming—how can it be?"

TAKE A DEEP BREATH

Did you know that when you take repeated deep breaths, your heart rate falls into sync? Deep breathing has long been the basis of relaxation practices like meditation and yoga. The deeper you breathe, the more oxygen you bring into every cell of your body, including your brain. When your brain is well oxygenated, you are able to think more clearly. Also, when you breathe deeply, your brain releases endorphins, chemicals that have a calming effect.

According to Harvard University, deep breathing can counter stress and its cousins anxiety and depression.[3] Have you noticed that when you feel stressed or anxious, you tend to take short, shallow breaths? Doing so only makes your stress worse. You might wonder how to breathe deeply. Try this: Breathe in through your nose and let your chest fill and your belly expand. If you want, hold in your breath

---

3   Harvard Health Publishing, Harvard Medical School, accessed April 3, 2022, https://www.health.harvard.edu/mind-and-mood/relaxation-techniques-breath-control-helps-quell-errant-stress-response.

for a count of three before you exhale through your mouth. Get in the habit of taking deep breaths during the day. Practice breathing when you feel stress coming on or you need to calm yourself. If you work at a desk, stand up and take ten deep breaths every few hours, or start your day in your favorite comfortable chair taking deep breaths while thinking affirming thoughts to start your day from a place of strength and contentment.

Deep breathing and its centering effects are a good metaphor for growing older. We are shifting into our age and accepting it rather than fighting it. When I was younger, I got in the habit of thinking a positive thought as I breathed in and releasing a negative thought as I breathed out. For example, when breathing in, I'd say "peace" (in my head or out loud), and breathing out I'd say "anxiety," which I would release with my breath. Or I would breathe in "strength" and breathe out "worry." It's not terribly original. You've probably done it too. But it's a good practice to remember to do. Besides, who doesn't need more calm in their life?

When trying yoga and intentional breathing, you might feel an emotional discharge of the worry, stress, and noise of everyday life. Sometimes, at the end of a yoga session I am crying, or I'm laughing, or I feel like falling asleep. It's a release of every thought that doesn't serve me, like one big exhale. With the great bonus of moving.

Find your yoga. Once you find a movement that fills you with passion, do it every day.

If you've already found your yoga, recommit to it. Yoga has helped me embrace my fifties. Like cooking, movement is self-expression. Maybe you always wanted to learn how to belly dance or line dance. Do it! Follow that urge. Listen to that young spirit inside of you that says, "Oooh. That sounds like fun!" If it feels like too big of a leap, take a step in between. For example, instead of jumping in and taking a belly dancing class, start by finding some live music that's coming to town and plan a night out with friends to go dancing, or take a drop-in Zumba class. Once you find your yoga and it sparks a passion, you've just created a way to stay healthy and add some new meaning to your life. Who knows? Maybe you have more than one yoga. If so, more power to you!

Finally, honor where you are at with movement. Take it day by day. Rome was not built in a day, and we were not meant to be built in a day either. If you've fallen out of the habit of being active, that's okay. Every day you get a chance to begin again. I encourage you to take a fresh look at what movement brings you joy. If it feels good and fills your spirit, then you are bound to keep doing it. Remove any kind of pressure, as in "I should go to the gym three days a week." If all that you can muster is going on Saturday after a long work week, that's just fine. If you keep it up, it will soon become a habit. Then, add movement as you go along. Consider simple, creative ways you can add movement to your days.

Maybe your mind is willing but your body is not. Again, take it slow and steady, and soon you will find that the two are in sync. It's okay to modify your workout. I mean, some days I simply don't feel like standing on my head! We have to honor our moods and our energy levels and find a balance between being gentle with ourselves and challenging ourselves.

As we age, we tend to feel more aches and pains. The body gets stiffer, thanks to less lubricating fluid inside aging joints, coupled with thinner cartilage. With age, bones get more brittle and don't heal as fast. The key is maintaining flexibility. If you can stretch for ten to fifteen minutes both morning and evening (do it while you are waking up with your favorite beverage, catching up on the news, or listening to your favorite podcast at night), you will have fewer aches and pains as you grow, according to the Cleveland Clinic.[4]

Okay, I hate to bring it up, but I have to.

> ## There's no getting around it when talking about loving and caring for our fiftysomething bodies—menopause!

The other night, I took a break from cooking to go out with my husband and one of our couple friends. I went to the extra effort of getting all dolled up. I put on a cocktail dress and spent time on my makeup, and I was happy with what I saw in the mirror. We arrived at the restaurant, and, not even a minute after taking my first bite of an appetizer and having a few sips of wine, I got a wicked hot flash. I'm talking about the ones that make you want to jump out of your skin. One layer, two layer, three layers all came off, and I was searching for something to make a fan. I grabbed the menu, and I hit my water glass, spilling water into my lap. (It's one way to cool down, but I don't recommend it!) At least I gave everyone at the table a good laugh.

Maybe you have a funny hot flash story to tell, so get together with girlfriends and tell it. 'Cuz all we can do is make light of it. If I'm not laughing about it, I'm crying, and I'd rather be laughing. I don't know about you, but I haven't found much of anything that helps. For me, I think there's a connection between alcohol and menopause. A friend of mine says that she thinks hot flashes are tied

---

[4] Cleveland Clinic, "Dealing with Common Aches and Pains as We Age with Dr. Donald Ford," accessed April 8, 2022, https://my.clevelandclinic.org/podcasts/health-essentials/dealing-with-common-aches-and-pains-as-we-age-with-dr-donald-ford.

to feeling nervous. Another woman I know says her hot flashes are like clockwork—occurring almost exactly seven minutes after she falls asleep, turning her bed into a torture chamber with repeated awakenings until she gets so exhausted she somehow sleeps through them. And what's up with the cold flash afterward?

According to the North American Menopause Society (NAMS), a cold chill often follows a hot flash, and a few women experience only the chill.[5] NAMS also says that hot flashes vary from woman to woman, and some women just have them for a total of six months (if that's you, I'm so jealous), while others have them as long as ten years (gawd, I'm so sorry).

Menopause is a natural part of aging, yet if it's disrupting your life, NAMS suggests that you explore prescription hormone therapy (for women who can take hormones safely), which is FDA approved and deemed safe (but not for women who have had breast, ovarian, or endometrial cancer). Some women who don't want to take hormones find relief with other medications. You can try a natural remedy, but there's not a lot of good evidence to support their effectiveness. If you are suffering, ask your doctor for a solution that's right for you. Whew! Now that we are done discussing hot flashes, let's cool down with a Yogurt Sundae.

---

5   North American Menopause Society, "Menopause FAQS: Hot Flashes," accessed April 4, 2022, https://www.menopause.org/for-women/menopause-faqs-hot-flashes.

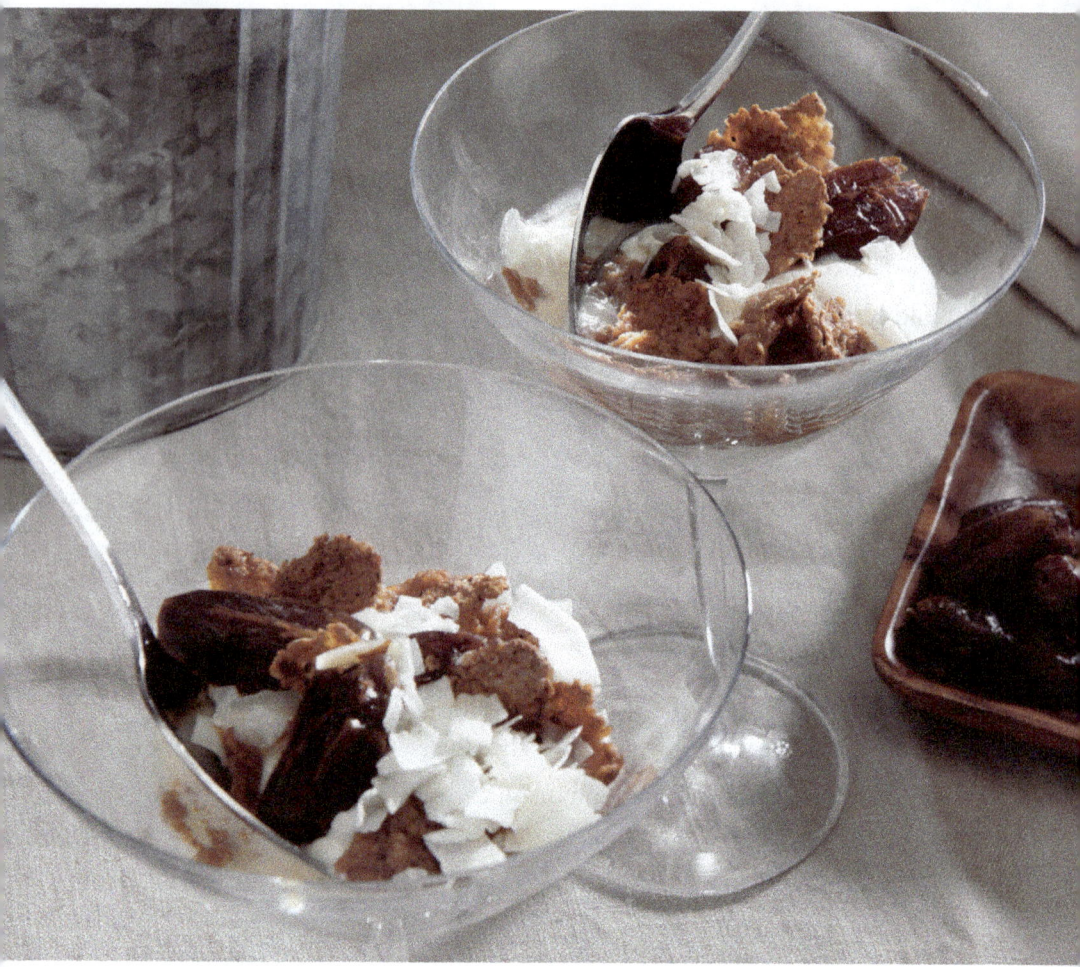

Yogurt Sundae

- 5 ounces yogurt, any flavor
- 3 dates
- ¼ cup protein flakes cereal
- 2 teaspoons dried coconut flakes

Layer yogurt and dates in a martini glass (I mean, we gotta have some fun). Top with cereal and coconut flakes. Enjoy!

Sadly, hot flashes are just one symptom of menopause. According to HealthCentral, the most common symptoms of menopause are hot flashes, night sweats (just hot flashes at night), insomnia, vaginal dryness, a lower libido, depression, anxiety, mood swings—oh my gosh, there's more—brain fog, and the urge to go number one a lot.[6] Wow. I'm sorry to drop that bomb if you are not quite fifty (or fifty-one, the average age menopause starts).

So here's a funny thought. Why do most of these symptoms have to do with being in bed? You can't sleep because hot flashes (or the urge to pee) wake you up; you have to work harder to be intimate with your partner (thanks to feeling dry down there or feeling depressed and wanting to cry your eyes out). It all makes you want to stay in bed. Sometimes I lie there awake and hold it because I don't want to get up and go. How lazy is that? I know the only way I'll get back to sleep is if I get up and go, but I try to wish it away. Dang you, dropping hormone levels!

If you are always going to the bathroom, doctors at HealthCentral suggest you cut back on soda, alcohol, and coffee (the latter will also help you sleep better) and get back in the habit of doing Kegel exercises (or start, if you never learned) to strengthen your pelvic floor muscles and help you avoid leakage. Yoga and Pilates are two activities that are great for creating a stronger pelvic floor. Just an FYI, if you do opt for hormone therapy, there's a good chance it will help restore your natural lubrication, along with other symptoms of menopause, according to HealthCentral. It's definitely a personal choice for every woman to make for herself with the help of her doctor.

Getting your menopause symptoms under control will help improve your sleep. Good sleep is so important to us feeling good as

---

[6] HealthCentral, "Let's Talk about Menopause," accessed April 4, 2022, https://www.healthcentral.com/condition/menopause.

we age. Studies show that sleep patterns change as we age. Before I had kids, I was an all-star sleeper, but that ended with new motherhood. You've likely heard all the downsides of poor sleep, so I won't get into them here. I'd rather encourage you to simply accept that your sleep patterns might change as you age. Do your best to set yourself up for good sleep, then accept those few extra wake ups during the night. Somehow, you will probably still have energy and a clear head to work and go about your life the next day.

Personally, I have had good luck with drinking a small cup of sleep-enhancing tea, like chamomile, about fifteen minutes before bed. I have also learned that we should adopt a soothing routine before bed, which includes avoiding screens, using low lighting, playing gentle music, and keeping our bedtime regular. When I exercise, I also tend to sleep better. Experts say that if you wake up in the middle of the night, it's best to get out of bed and do something quiet, like reading, until you feel sleepy again. Also, try not to look at the clock when you wake up during the night. Everyone has their own way to promote sleep, so I encourage you to find what works for you.

Lastly, we can't talk about menopause and aging without discussing metabolism, which drops as we age. Partly because we lose muscle mass as we age, which computes to burning fewer calories. And if you think you've gained more weight around your middle, you can blame our little friend menopause for that. According to Mayo Clinic, hormonal changes make it more likely that you will gain weight around your gut more quickly than other places, like your thighs or hips.[7] But you don't have to accept the dreaded belly bulge. We are wise, wonderful women who know our own bodies.

---

[7] Mayo Clinic, "Menopause Weight Gain: Stop the Middle Age Spread," accessed April 11, 2022, https://www.mayoclinic.org/healthy-lifestyle/womens-health/in-depth/menopause-weight-gain/art-20046058.

Remember, if you don't rev up your metabolism, it won't rev you up! Just another Maria-ism to live by.

With a newfound commitment to moving every day and finding your own yoga, you have the power within you to maintain a weight that's healthy for you and design life habits that benefit you. Even if your mind says it's too late for you, it's not. As an older woman, you can change your mindset and take back some of your youthful spirit. You can recommit each and every day to having the body you want—not what others deem right for you but the weight and movement that makes you feel good in your own skin. It's part of the power of being fifty-plus!

In the next chapter, I'll share daily habits that help me say no to the slowdown of metabolism, like jump-starting a lighter diet with a cleanse, eating tips to maintain a healthy weight, and some light but delicious lunches made from fresh ingredients. C'mon, it's a fresh start!

TREE POSE

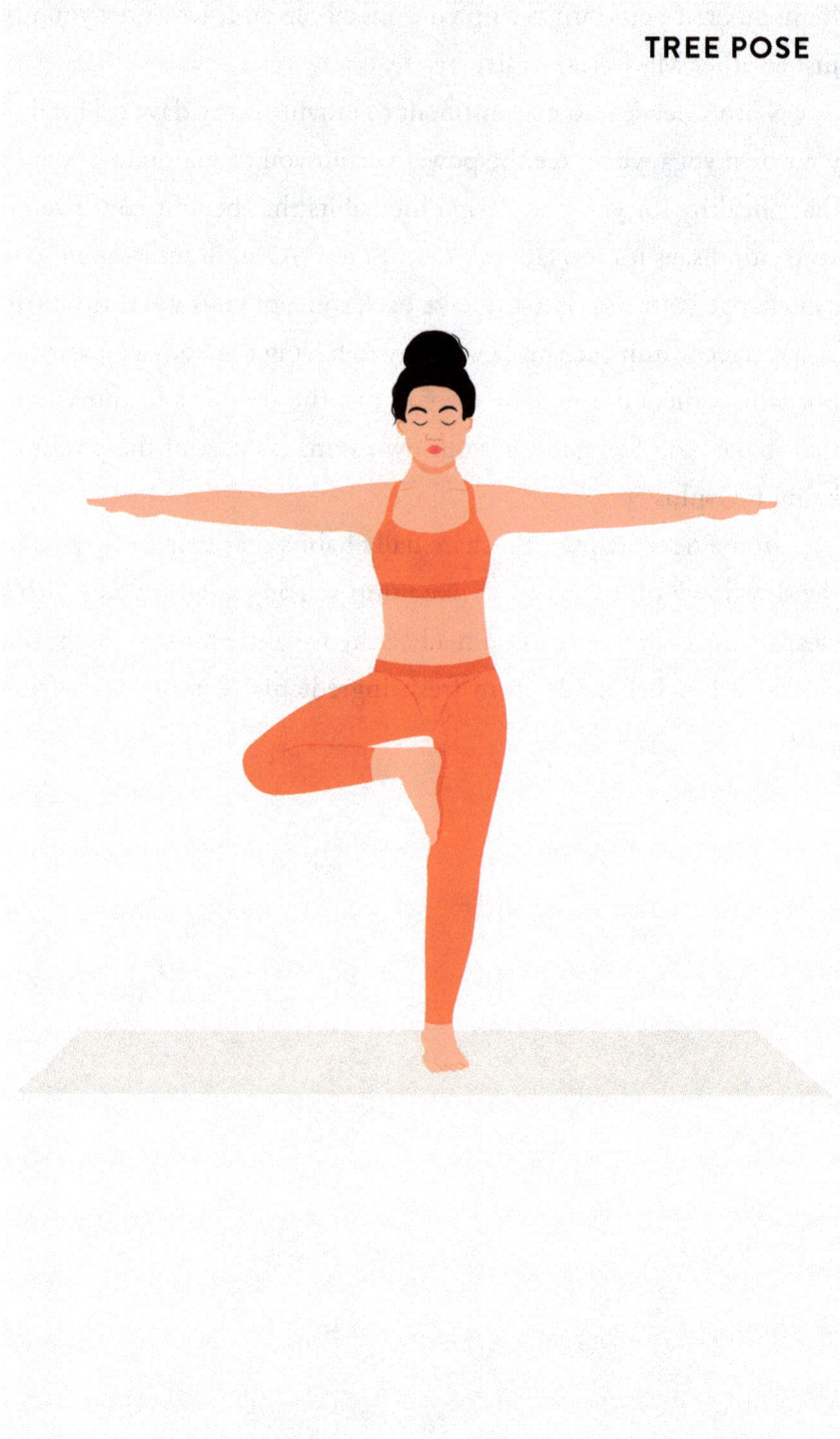

MOVE WITH MEANING

It's time to rise up from child's pose and stand tall in tree pose. I invite you to come into your own and find your balance. Tree pose is often used to muster up strength before you move ahead with a more challenging pose. Trees link us to both the earth and the heavens. Feel the steadiness of the ground while you embrace your own spirituality, however you define it, and wisdom. Gather your strength to move forward and face the challenges in your life.

1. Stand steady on two feet. Shift your weight to your dominant foot and keep your leg straight without locking your knee.
2. Lift your other foot and place the sole of your foot, as high as you can, on the inner thigh of your supporting leg.
3. Gain balance by placing equal pressure on your resting and standing feet.
4. Stretch your arms out to your sides at shoulder height.
5. Spend a few minutes in tree pose meditating on gratitude for your body and all the support it has given you through the years. Inhale deeply and say, "I am strong. I respect my body." Exhale and say, "I release shame about my [fill in the blank with your neglected or tortured body part]." Consider how you view your fiftysomething body and set an intention for something you'd like to achieve by the end of this book. Maybe it's losing weight or accepting your

current weight. Maybe it's about improving your diet or adding more movement. Maybe it's gaining self-confidence or letting go of regrets. Repeat your own personal, positive mantra as you breathe in and breathe out until you feel some peace around your body and its beautiful, intricate ability to carry you through your days.

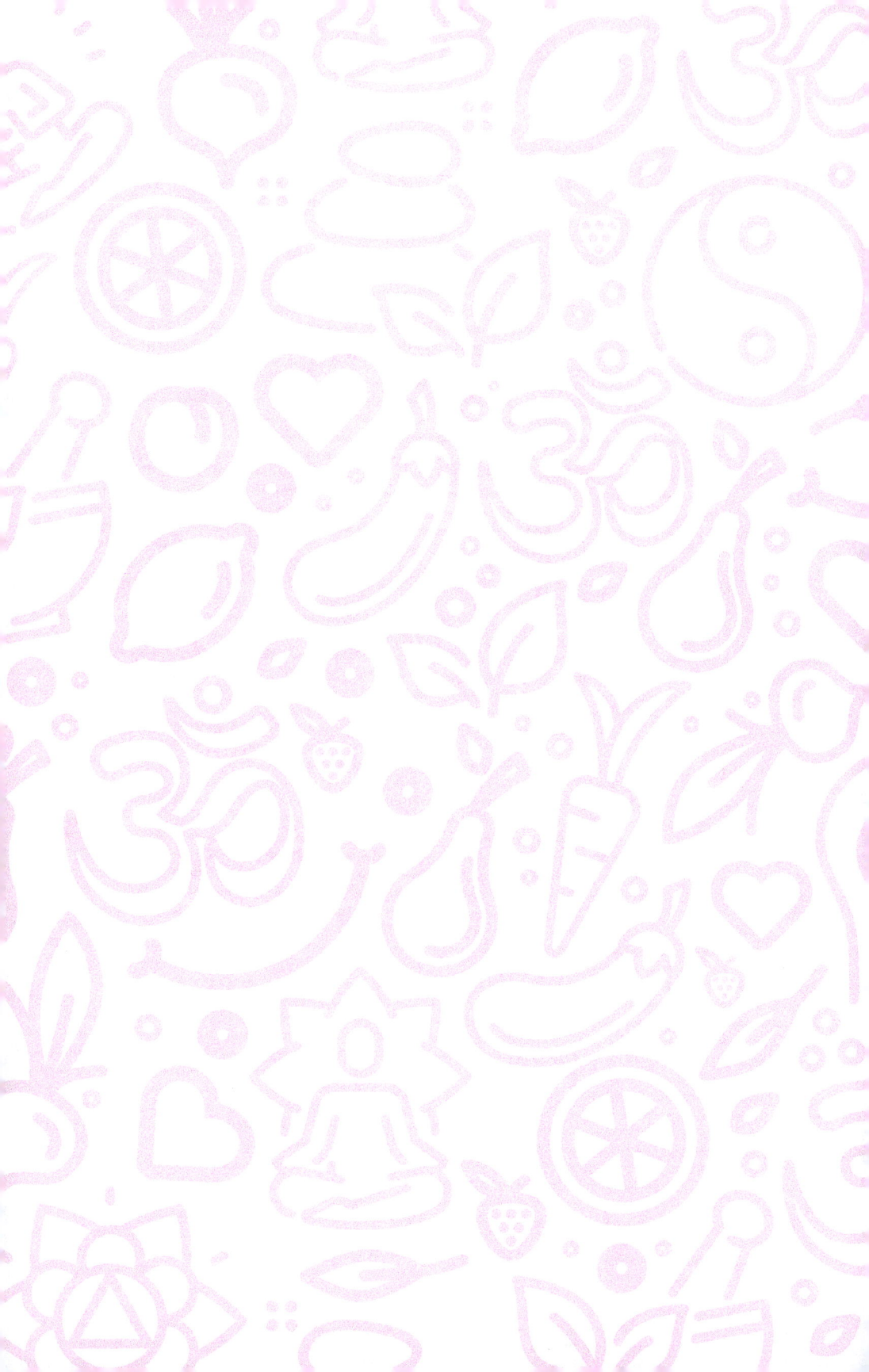

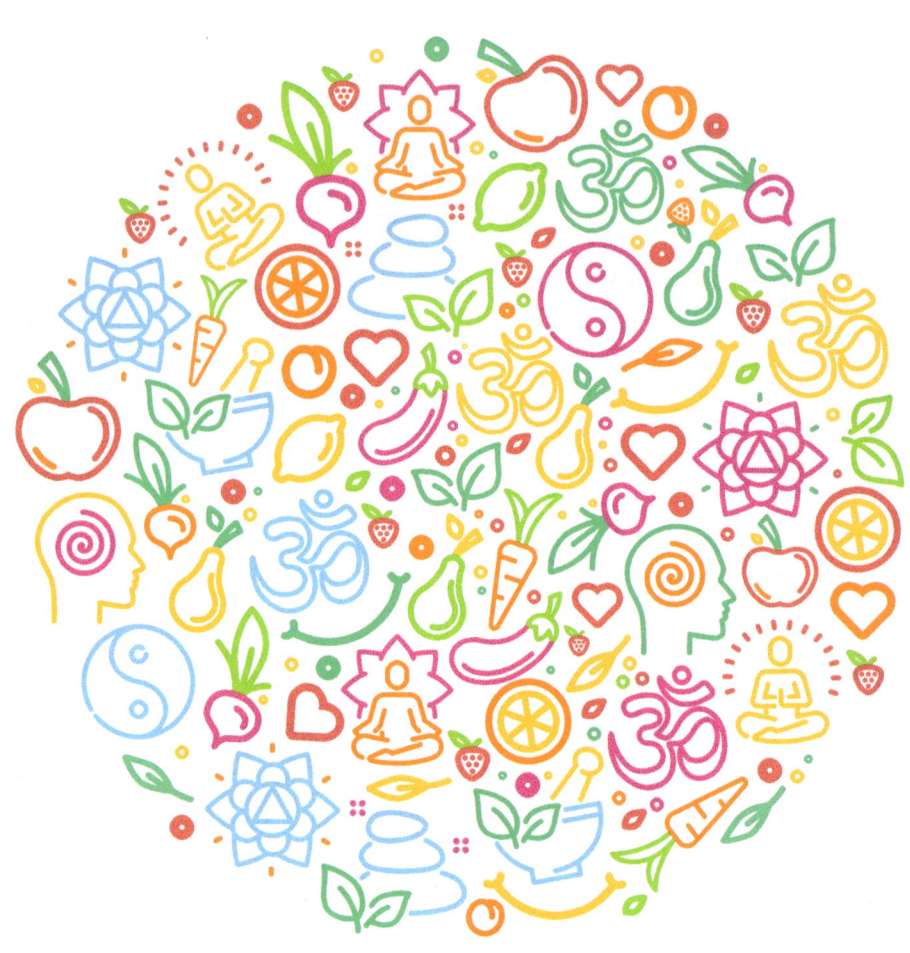

CHAPTER 3

A Fresh Start

Freshen up with Pear Brie Salad

A h, summer. My favorite time of year for one of my favorite activities—going to the farmers market. I can feel excitement building from the minute I get out of bed, thinking of all the fresh vegetables and fruits that I'll find and dreaming about what I'll make with them. On Saturdays, the indoor market near my house is packed, and I have to fight against a current of people, but I don't mind. I get the biggest wagon I can find, and I go from booth to booth, sniffing fruit, inspecting vegetables, and chatting with workers from the various farms. I feel like a fancy pioneer woman as I search for the perfect shallot or the ripest Jersey tomato.

There's something about going on my own and getting to move at my own pace that makes all the sights and sounds simply delicious. I relish in the scent of fresh Georgia peaches and celebrate finding my favorite jarred pickles. I can't resist a perfectly seasoned dill pickle! I select a rainbow of vegetables, including dark-green romaine, perfect for one of my all-time tasty recipes, Pear Brie Salad. It's a perfect lunch. For me, the farmers market feels like a fresh start, a reset at the end of a long week. It's a type of meditation that centers me by letting me lose myself in the simplest purpose of life, namely feeding myself and my family healthy food.

Pear Brie Salad

1 head romaine lettuce, chopped
1 pear, chopped
¼ cup chopped walnuts
3 (2-inch) chunks of Brie cheese

For lemon vinaigrette:
¼ cup olive oil
½ teaspoon salt
Juice of 1 lemon

Combine all ingredients except those for vinaigrette. Prepare vinaigrette and mix well. Toss over salad.

Until I can plant my own garden—something that's high on my bucket list—I am content with these regular trips to the farmers market and planting a few vegetables in pots. After all, I didn't go the country-girl route. I'm a city girl. But I do dream about a little Italian garden out back with tomatoes, garlic, lettuce, arugula, basil, and oregano. I think fresh tomatoes are what help Italians live long lives.

When I cook, I like to think of the meal as a canvas. I use colors that complement and excite. We can create a mood simply by choosing the right combination of ingredients and presenting them in a pleasing way. One of my habits is trying to eat foods as close to

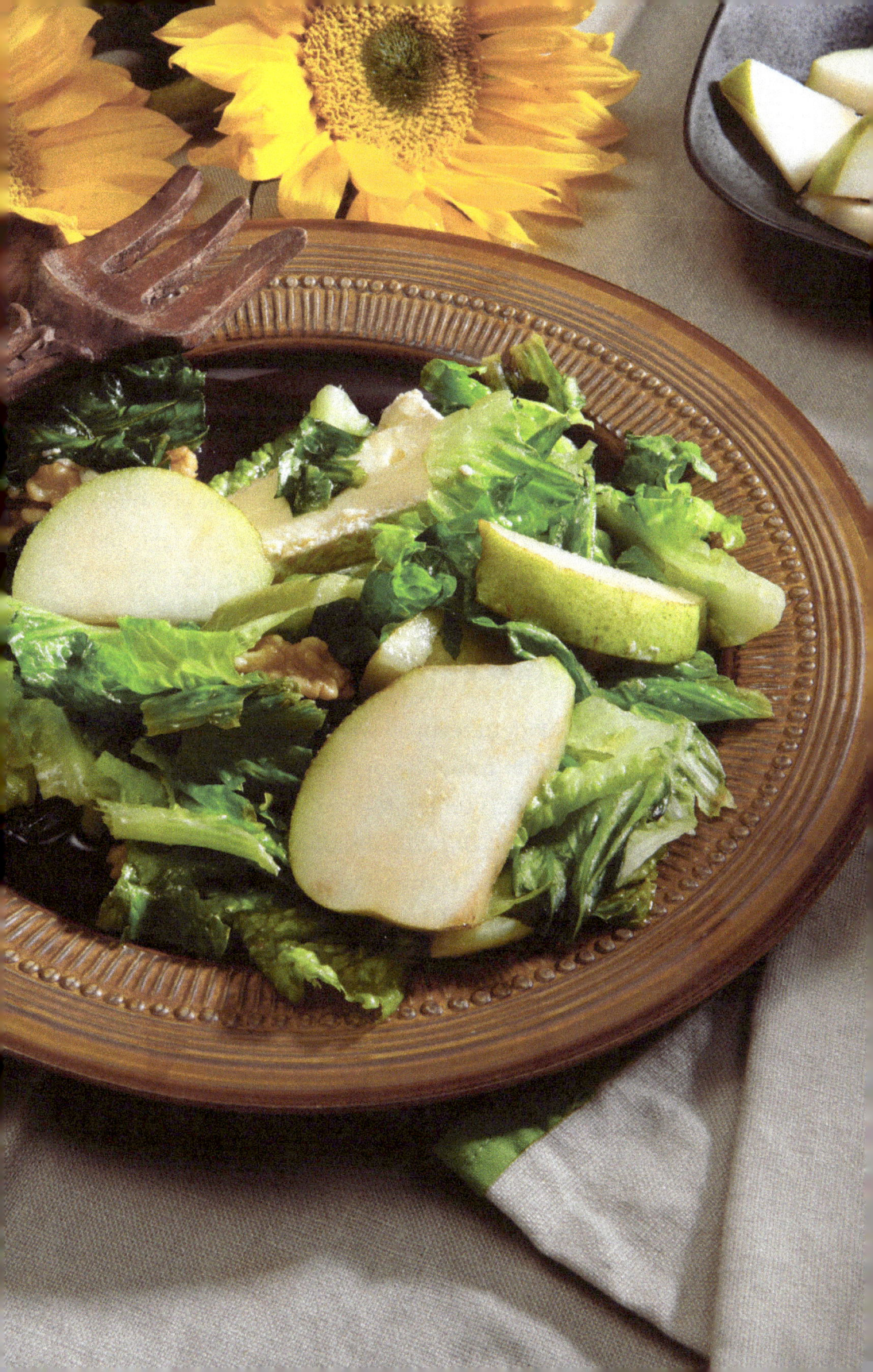

nature as they come. I notice that I feel better when I steer clear of foods that are processed or are high in sugar or unhealthy saturated fat. When I eat a balance of healthy vegetables, fruits, and clean meat that's not fried or breaded, I feel more energy.

This habit is especially important for lunchtime, in my opinion. Heavy foods like pizza, which are full of carbs and sugar, just make me extra hungry for dinner. That's why I like to keep it fresh and light for lunch. If I eat too light, it doesn't sustain me, and I get hungry. I make sure to include ingredients that provide some oomph, like nuts, lighter cheeses, lean meats, and fish. Whenever I can, I try to balance fats, carbohydrates, and proteins in my meals. This habit of eating a fulfilling yet lighter lunch helps me maintain a healthy weight, and snacks between meals keep my blood sugar steady.

SHOULD I BUY ORGANIC?

There's a lot of debate over whether or not there are health benefits to eating organic foods. It's best to turn to scientific studies for the answer, like the one published in the *British Journal of Nutrition* that reviewed 343 studies comparing organic and conventional foods to find common themes.[8] Here's what the researchers found:

- In general, there are not significant differences in nutrition between organic and nonorganic foods.
- However, when it comes to antioxidants (natural

---

[8] *British Journal of Nutrition*, "Higher Antioxidant and Lower Cadmium Concentrations and Lower Incidence of Pesticide Residues in Organically Grown Crops: A Systemic Literature Review and Meta-analyses," accessed on April 12, 2022, https://pubmed.ncbi.nlm.nih.gov/24968103/.

ingredients in fruits and vegetables that have been proven to protect the cells in our bodies from free radicals [these molecules may increase the risk for cancer, heart disease, and other diseases]), organic crops have a substantially higher amount.
- Pesticide residues were four times higher in conventional versus organic fruits and vegetables.
- Toxic metals were significantly higher in conventional versus organic crops.

Eating organic versus conventional is a personal choice. Since organic food tends to cost more, it's also a financial choice. I try to buy organic whenever I can, but sometimes I pick and choose just certain foods that are organic so that I can keep my food budget in check. Have you heard of the dirty dozen? It's the twelve fruits and vegetables (strawberries, spinach, kale, grapes, etc.) that have the highest concentrations of pesticides. Buying locally, like at the farmers market, can mean less pesticides since the food sold is often from small farmers who don't need to heavily preserve their crops to ship them across the country. Some people choose to buy organic meat products because environmental pollutants, like dioxins, are stored in the fat of animals.[9] Do what feels most comfortable for you.

---

[9] World Health Organization, "Dioxins and Their Effects on Human Health," accessed April 12, 2022, https://www.who.int/news-room/fact-sheets/detail/dioxins-and-their-effects-on-human-health.

If you feel like your metabolism has taken a dive off the deep end, like we talked about in chapter 2, there's a good chance you are struggling to maintain a healthy weight. I have a few eating tips to help with that. One is replacing calories with spices. The tastier something is, the more satisfied you feel after eating it. Other tips include eating slowly and stopping regularly to enjoy the conversation with your family and friends between bites. It takes a while for our hunger signals to stop chiming once we start eating. If we eat fast, we might keep eating because we think we are still hungry, but really we are getting full. And focusing on good company at a meal is the best flavoring of all! Another tip to avoid weight gain is using dressings or sauces lightly. It's an easy place to cut back on calories. My Tuna Pasta Salad is a great example of a light sauce that packs a punch.

I want to share with you a huge tip for maintaining your weight. It has to do with what I call calorie amnesia. Calorie amnesia is brought on by feeling so great after exercising that you think you burned endless calories. Put simply, it's thinking, "I can eat whatever I want today. It's all fine because I worked out!" More than likely the calories you reward yourself with will outweigh the calories you burned, even if you ran five miles. It seems to me that you'd be better off dancing around the kitchen while you cook up a healthy meal than you would be taking that run and then eating a fried-chicken dinner. I'm not advocating that you stop moving—no way—just that you keep it in perspective and maybe exercise for fitness rather than weight loss. If you've had a good workout and you are feeling hungry, try my decadent yet light Salmon Chowder for lunch.

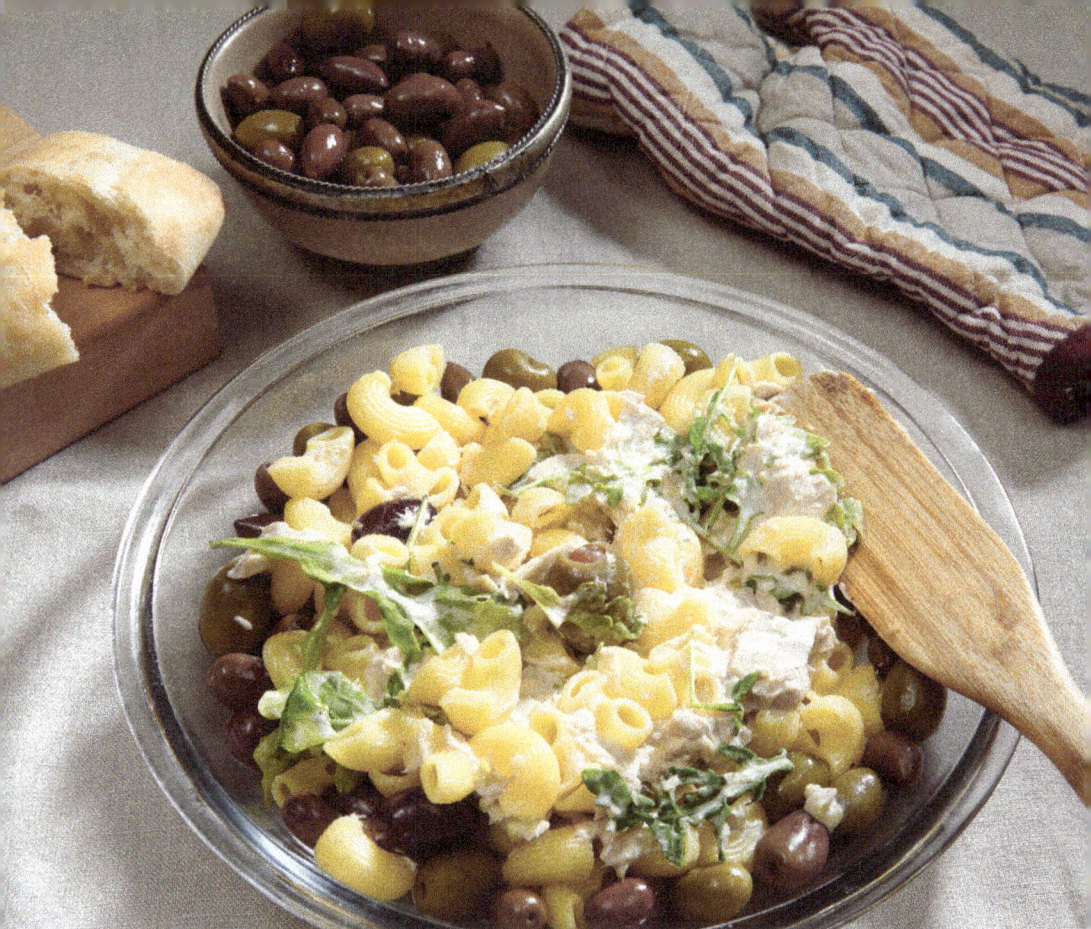

Tuna Pasta Salad

> ½ pound cooked pasta
> ¾ cup light mayonnaise
> ¼ cup light ranch dressing
> 1 can tuna, drained
> ½ cup arugula
> 1 cup assorted olives as garnish

Combine all ingredients in a bowl except for the olives. Arrange olives along edge of bowl as a decorative border. Enjoy!

Salmon Chowder

5 ounces salmon fillet, cut into cubes
1 (10-ounce) box chicken broth
1 teaspoon rosemary
1 teaspoon olive oil
1 garlic clove, thinly sliced
Salt and pepper, to taste
¼ cup cream cheese
¼ cup cornstarch
¼ cup warm water
¼ cup shredded cheddar cheese
¼ cup oyster crackers

Place oil and garlic in a saucepan and sauté. Meanwhile, combine cornstarch and water in a small bowl and mix well. Add chicken broth, salmon cubes, cream cheese, and rosemary and mix well. Allow to boil, then simmer. Turn off the heat and sprinkle in cheddar cheese and allow it to melt. Top with oyster crackers and get ready for something good!

To avoid calorie amnesia, stay awake! In other words, be mindful about what you put in your mouth. Make eating a sit-down activity and really experience your meal. We've all eaten something while we were preoccupied, reaching for another bite only to find that it's all gone. Staying aware while we eat adds up to feeling more satisfied and helps us resist eating blindly.

I want to add a plug for healthy oils. With each year that passes, we need to add more healthy oils, like olive oil, fish, nuts, and avocados, to our meals. Healthy oils feed our brains, and they are mighty warriors

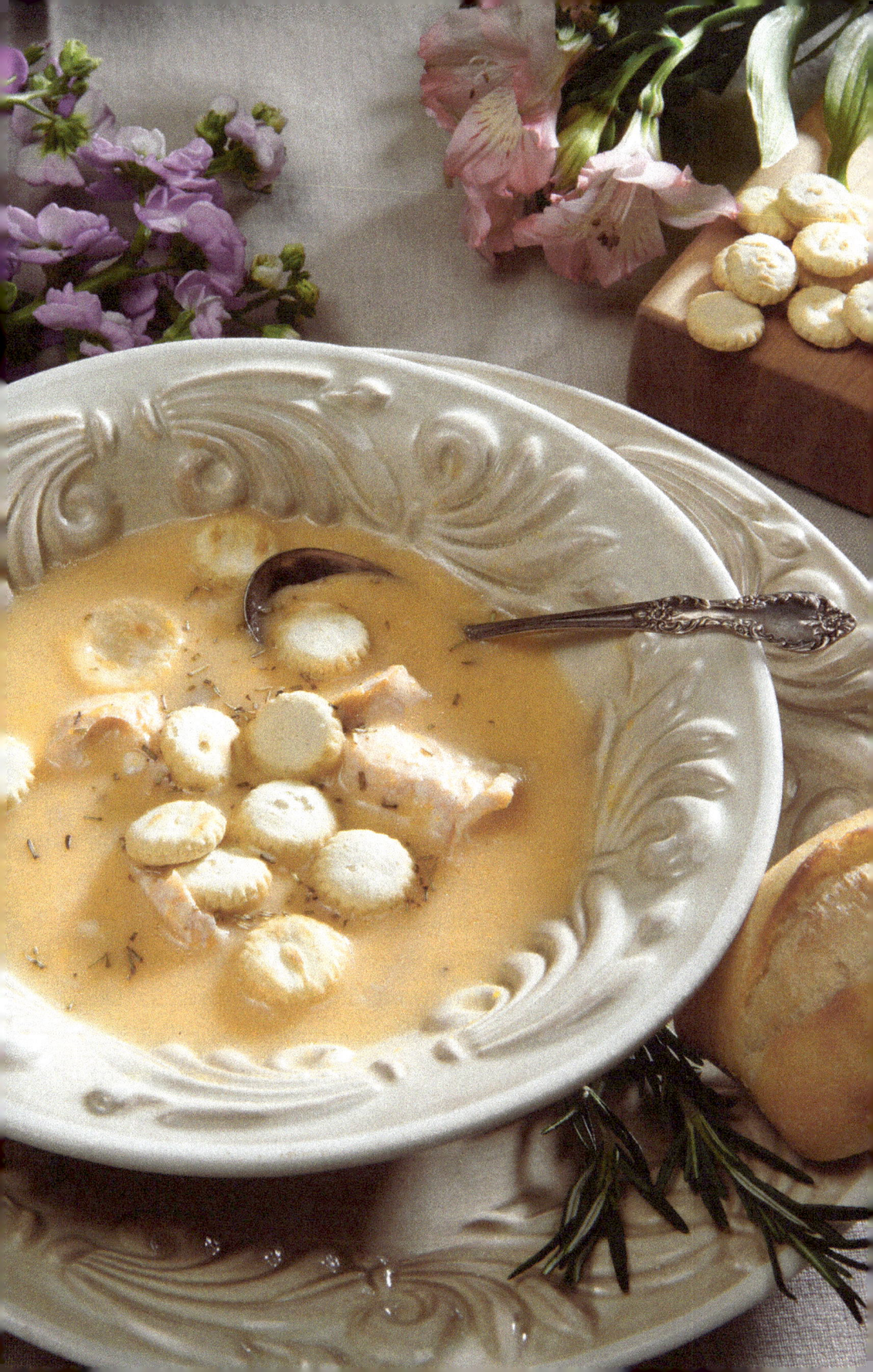

against Alzheimer's disease and other forms of brain degeneration. We Italians love olive oil, and we tend to start nearly every meal with a splash in the pan or in our salads. There's wisdom stored in different cultures, and cooking with olive oil is one that the Italian heritage shares with the world. It's funny to me how it flies in the face of low-fat fad diets of the past. In college, I would chastise my mother for using too much olive oil. It just goes to show that each of us needs to devise a diet that fits us, our heritage, and our lifestyle, driven by our own internal wisdom and innate needs. Personally, I like my food salty and spicy with a lot of color from fruits and vegetables, some starch, and a nice amount of healthy fat.

Sometimes, even when I do everything right, I still feel like it's hard to maintain my chosen weight. Or I feel sluggish. That's when I consider a cleanse. Cleansing is an ancient practice that dates back to 2000 BC. The way I do a cleanse is nothing to record in the history books, but it gives me a fresh start. Usually, a day of cleansing is just right for me, maybe two. Sometimes, I mix things up and replace a meal a day with a cleansing drink. My favorite way to cleanse is with smoothies and teas that infuse my body with healthy ingredients, but that wasn't always the case. I remember doing a tomato cleanse with friends in college, which ultimately led to Bloody Marys! After a fun night out—a little too fun if you know what I mean—is a perfect time to do a cleanse.

Check with your doctor to make sure a mild cleanse is okay for you. The goal of a cleanse is to flush toxins out of your body. Start by picking high-quality, preferably organic, fruits and veggies, like blueberries, apples, bananas, watermelon, mangos, spinach, kale, and chard. Follow your gut, literally, to decide if you want to keep it extra light by blending with water and ice only or if you want to add a little oomph with an unsweetened milk alternative or coconut water. Even adding plain yogurt to a detox smoothie is just fine in my book, like I do with my Kale Smoothie.

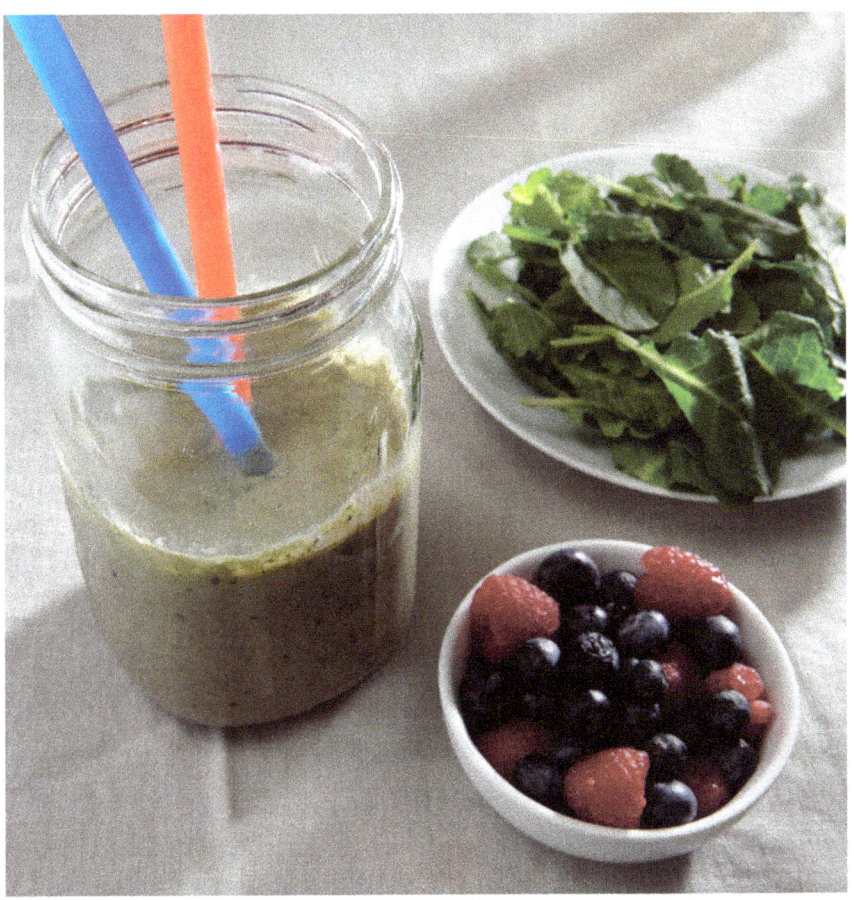

Kale Smoothie

½ cup frozen blueberries or raspberries

1 cup kale or spinach leaves

5 ounces low-fat vanilla or plain yogurt

½ cup almond milk

½ cup cranberry juice

2 ice cubes

Puree in blender or juicer. Sip and enjoy.

For an extra detox kick, include an herb or two that's known to detox your gallbladder, liver, and intestines, such as dandelion root, milk thistle, or turmeric. (Turmeric, and its main ingredient, curcumin, is thought to be a huge anti-inflammatory, so if you have diabetes, arthritis, asthma, or another inflammatory disease, give turmeric a special place in your kitchen and in your heart.[10]) If it's easier, buy herbs in capsule form and simply break apart the capsule and dump them in with your other smoothie ingredients. Also, pick up some garlic and cilantro and add them for extra tang and detoxification. Sip green tea throughout the day for even more detoxifying action. A personal favorite tea of mine to drink while cleansing is chamomile tea with cilantro and mint. I believe that tea and herbs are a cornerstone of good health.

The great thing about cleansing and eating real, whole food that nourishes your body is the energy that it gives you. Some people might look great on the outside, but they eat junk or starve themselves and they don't feel good on the inside. Feeling good inside trumps looking good outside every time. Yet the two are connected. When we eat well, it often shows in our clear eyes, bright face, and the confident way we carry ourselves. We know we are taking care of ourselves, and that's self-love. When you look in the mirror, I hope you like what you see. You are beautiful. Everyone has beauty. See if you can spot your internal glow in the glint in your eye or the healthy color in your cheeks! It comes from treating your body well and relishing in the love and support that you get from self-care and care from others.

While inner beauty rules, it also feels good to love our outer selves by wearing clothes that we feel good in, having a hairstyle that suits

---

10   "Mayo Clinic Q&A: Turmeric's Anti-inflammatory Properties May Relieve Arthritis Pain," accessed April 22, 2022, https://newsnetwork.mayoclinic.org/discussion/mayo-clinic-q-and-a-turmerics-anti-inflammatory-properties-may-relieve-arthritis-pain/.

us, and applying makeup in a way that enhances our natural features. We get to feel good on the inside *and* feel good on the outside! In chapter 10, I dive into how to dress your best so you feel good about yourself out in the world. Personal grooming and care is an expression of self-respect, just like eating well and exercising regularly.

Every now and then, we need a fresh start, so I hope some of the ideas in this chapter were helpful. You've been around the block millions of times, and you are smart, so many of these ideas are probably just reminders, and if you are like me, you need plenty of those these days! Coming up, I share some of the healthy habits that I have integrated into my life that help me maintain a weight that I feel good at, which nourishes a healthy dose of self-acceptance and celebration in being fabulous at fifty-plus. Let's lighten up and love ourselves!

LOVING LIFE AT 50+

DOWNWARD DOG

MOVE WITH MEANING

You were standing tall in tree pose, and now it's time to come to the mat and get ready to work with downward dog. This is my favorite yoga pose because its deep stretch with arms out in front gives me the sense of flying. It looks like it would be simple to do, but it takes some effort, and it works your whole body. With this pose, you are renewing your strength. Feel your own power radiating up from your hands and your feet as you face the difficulty of this position.

1. Get on all fours, like our friendly canine friends.
2. Rise up on your hands and feet, with your hands out in front of you and your feet behind you, bending at the middle. Feel the stretch in your legs and back.
3. Rest your heels on the floor and make sure your ears are in line with your upper arms. Let your head relax.
4. Hold the pose for as long as you can as you breathe deeply. Muster up the courage to meditate on your own personal power. What makes you feel strong? What are you proud of? What defines you as a person? What traits help you face your fears? Let the positive answers fill you and give you strength. Also, consider a few habits you can start or reinstate to enhance your inner glow.
5. When you feel a bit spent from holding the pose, come down to your hands and knees and release your breath.

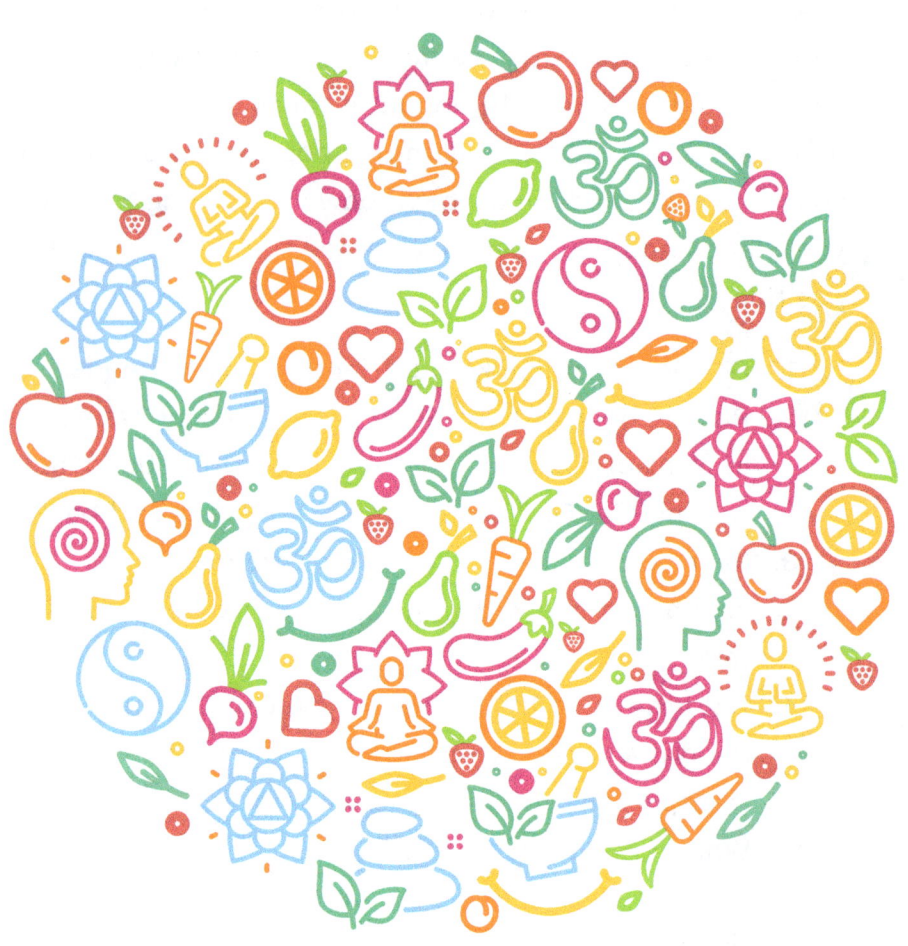

CHAPTER 4

Lighten Up
Keep Things Spicy with Cinnamon Popcorn

My maternal grandmother took great pride in her cooking, and she wanted to make sure we learned how to cook like old-world Italians. I remember one of her lessons in particular, which still makes me laugh today. I was in my midtwenties, and I was home for Thanksgiving. Mind you, alongside the turkey we always served homemade manicotti—a family tradition.

My grandmother, whom we call Nana, decided that it was high time that my sister and I learned how to make homemade pasta. If you've ever tried, you know that it's not easy. It demands patience, something we didn't have much of at the time. Instead of staying on task, we were getting silly and making a floury mess of everything. Nana was getting really annoyed. We Italians are particular about our traditions, and we can have a hot temper. Suddenly, she stopped rolling out the dough and looked at us with a stern face and said, "You college grads don't know a darn thing!" We doubled over in laughter, which only made her madder until she refused to go on. That phrase became a saying that my sister and I have used in hilarious iterations hundreds of times with each other.

I never did learn how to make homemade pasta—I just never had the time or, I'll admit, the patience. But I did teach my oldest daughter, Alyssa, to make lasagna in preschool. My mother taught me, so I taught her, keeping at least some of those old-world traditions alive. She still makes it today. And in my house, you have to serve it with a romaine-lettuce salad with balsamic vinegar, oil, salt, and pepper. My sister uses garlic pepper for a tasty twist. If you get iceberg instead of romaine, it's a cardinal sin.

Nana is behind all the Italian recipes that I've gathered over the years. They've been passed down from my mother, who scribbled them on index cards—God forbid I lose one!—stemming from thousands of meals served up over generations of Italian families.

Nana was onto something with her measured life and methods. Maintaining a healthy weight is all about moderation and establishing a few healthy habits that guide most of your days. I know it sounds boring. But it can be so, so satisfying. Routines give our life structure—just like breathing does—and best yet, when we stick to them most of the time, we get to break out once in a while for some fun! Snacks are part of this breaking out for me, and I like to keep things spicy when it comes to snacks, like with my Spicy Cinnamon Popcorn. Delicious.

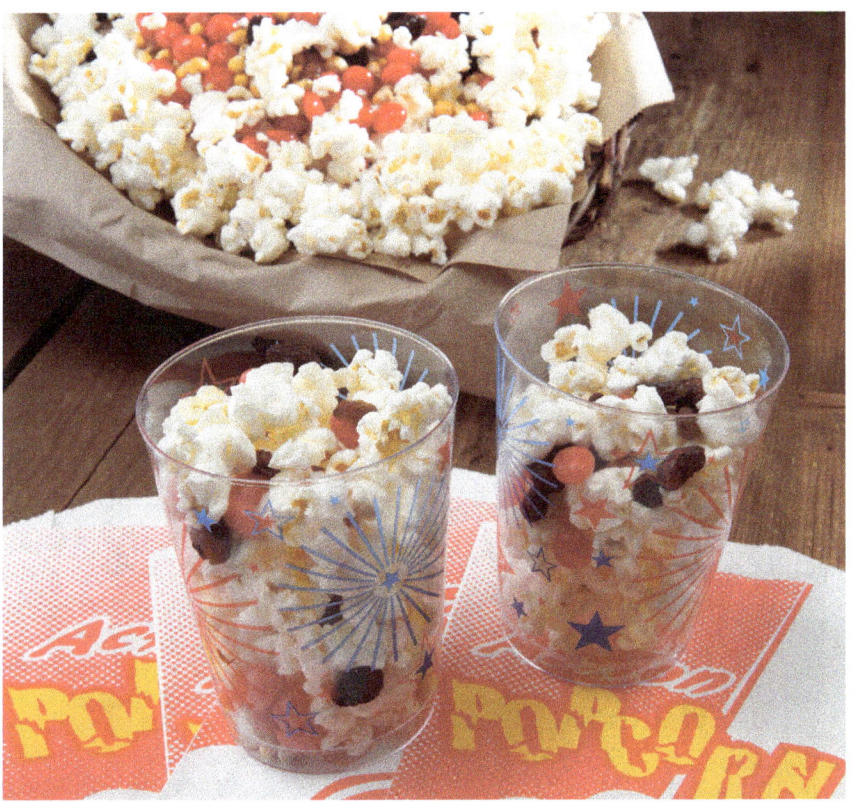

Spicy Cinnamon Popcorn

> 3 cups air-popped popcorn
>
> 1 teaspoon coconut oil
>
> 3 teaspoons cinnamon candies
>
> 3 teaspoons raisins
>
> ½ teaspoon chili pepper

Toss and enjoy.

Part of eating moderately for me is serving up smaller portions. I'm not going to give up my favorite rich dishes completely, but I will eat less of them. I love a glass of wine, but I resist having more than a glass or two most of the time. (I do like a good party now and then, so I save up my drink tickets!) I've also shifted my focus from how I look to how I feel and how I can bring the most meaning into my life. By doing things that make me happy, like spending time with my family (in the final chapter, you'll go along with me and my family on our trip to Italy), cooking delicious meals, watching football games, and doing yoga, I feel happier and more satisfied with my life. Feeling satisfied with my days keeps me from overeating. When life itself is gratifying, there's no empty hole inside that needs filling up.

The biggest willpower boost is cheerfulness.

Knowing my habits and keeping them top of mind helps me stay on track with my weight. I've struggled with weight much of my life. I've tried fad diets and succeeded, then failed too many times to count. I've tried starving myself, but that just sets me up for failure. I've learned from my mistakes. I no longer believe that staying hungry will keep me thin and lead to happiness, like I did when I was young. Now, I eat moderately and try to move every single day. When hunger comes, I welcome it and heed its call as a healthy signal from my body. I think, "My body wants food, so I better feed it."

Likely, you have your own habits to help you maintain a healthy weight. If you haven't ever sat down and written them out, I encourage you to do so. There's something magical about putting your personal philosophy for a healthy life on paper. Have you ever noticed that? If you write a goal down and stick it on the fridge, mirror, or computer where you can see it every day, somehow it magically gets fulfilled. Like it's granted by a fairy godmother. Poof! Of course, I don't think it's magic—it's more likely keeping it top of mind and consciously and subconsciously moving toward it—but whatever's behind it, it works. (In chapter 5, we'll do a deep dive into the power of journaling.) For inspiration, I'm sharing my habits for healthy eating and living. They are not groundbreaking, but if you stick to them, you will feel lighter.

MARIA'S HABITS FOR A HEALTHY WEIGHT

- **Watch your portions**. Eat the foods you want, just less of them!

- **Resist skipping meals**. Skipping meals makes you famished, which sends your blood sugar diving and causes you to overeat.

- **Eat on a schedule of breakfast, snack, lunch, snack, dinner**. It gives you a lot of chances to eat, and it keeps your blood sugar levels nice and steady.

- **Calories count, so count them**. Don't go crazy—just keep a loose count in your head or your journal. I've learned that eating roughly 1,200 to 1,500 calories a day is a good goal for myself as a woman.

- **Don't let the scale rule you**. The scale is just one form of measurement on how well you are doing. Gauge your success in other ways, like how your clothes fit, how good you feel, and whether or not you are moving every day.

Did you notice that I didn't say avoid carbs? I know limiting carbohydrates like bread and pasta is a big part of most weight-management plans. I get that, but hey, I'm Italian. What did you expect? It's almost sacrilegious to tell a 100 percent Italian not to eat pasta or bread! But

I have learned to eat less of it. I can pass on the bread and just eat the pasta, as my grandfather instructed my Nana to do at every single meal we ever shared. Poor Nana. She should've gotten feisty with him like she did with me when we were making pasta from scratch!

In a nutshell, when I'm trying to maintain my weight or lose a few pounds—never ever with the goal of getting stick thin, mind you—I am thoughtful about using less oil, meat, and, the saddest of all, bread. Yet this simple goal helps me lighten things up. Most of my recipes are lower in unhealthy fat, meat, and carbs, so hopefully they will help you lighten up, too, if that's something you want to do. (If putting on weight is what you need, then go full Italian with lots of healthy oils, nuts, seeds, whole grains, and yummy desserts.)

I like to say, "Eat until you are satisfied, not until you are stuffed." Sometimes you have to wait a bit to see if you are full. As I've said before, when you eat slowly, you will start feeling full before the end of your meal and stop before you are stuffed. When you feel satiated, you're more apt to put your fork down. Have you noticed that when you're eating and you get interrupted by a phone call, when you sit back down you're not hungry for your meal anymore? It's like that. Managing your appetite is more important than counting calories in my book.

I also don't believe in denying myself certain foods. My infamous motto is "Indulge or you'll bulge," which I discuss in its full glory in chapter 9. What I mean by this is that if you label foods as forbidden, you will fixate on them. Trust me, I know this from experience. The more you deny yourself, or try to control yourself, the worse it gets, and it can lead to binge eating. After all, we are humans, not robots. So when I have a craving, I feed it.

First, I recognize it as a craving and not hunger. That helps me stay ahead of the urge to overeat. Seeing it as a craving allows me to ask myself if I am feeding my feelings or if it's just a simple craving.

Knowing my motivation helps me give in just a little and not too much. I say, "A taste of honey is *not* worse than none at all!" Even a small piece of chocolate can satisfy. If you have a favorite candy bar and you spread it out over three days, you get to enjoy what you love without putting on unwanted pounds. It can be an indulgent snack. I love snacks that feel a wee bit indulgent, like my Fruit Smoothie with raspberry sorbet.

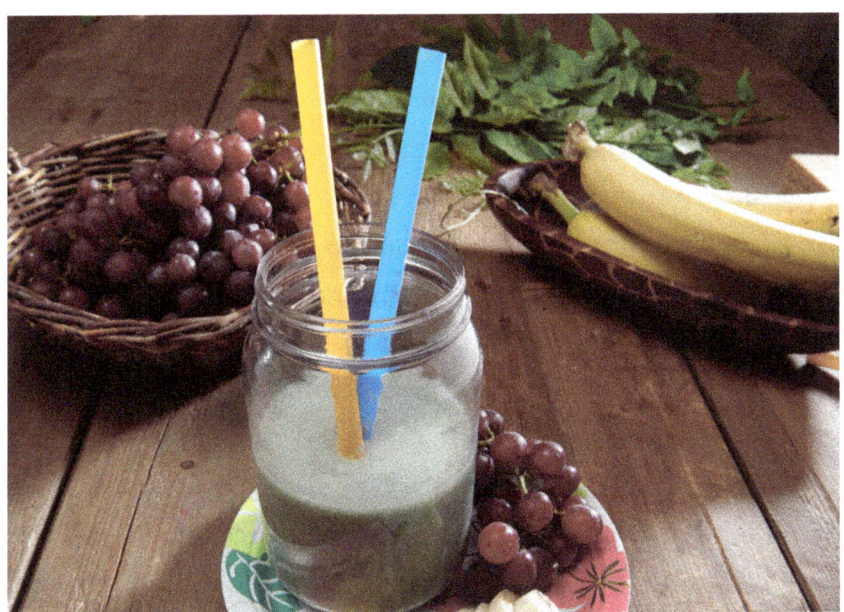

Fruit Smoothie

- 1 ripened banana
- ½ cup raspberry sorbet
- 2 ice cubes
- ½ cup almond milk
- ½ cup water
- 3 teaspoons whey protein

Puree in blender or juicer.

As I said, I've always struggled with my weight. In college, I went a little crazy counting calories and limiting what I ate. I know I'm not alone in this. I've talked to several women who fell into this trap, fueled by the fear of the freshman fifteen. While it wasn't a full-blown eating disorder, this dabbling was fairly common back in my day at college in the late '80s. Recently, I read that women in their fifties are at risk for eating disorders, which surprised me. According to an article in AARP, nearly 13 percent of American women who are fifty-plus struggle with an eating disorder, and a whopping 60 percent of us say that our weight and shape has a negative effect on our lives.[11]

This statistic makes two things crystal clear: As women, we need to have balance in our lives, and we have to be gentle with ourselves. If we restrict our diet and deny ourselves certain foods, we set ourselves up for failure. There's also the flip side to this: getting obsessed with healthy eating and exercise. Extremes in life are never good in my book. I say, if you want to treat yourself when you are out with friends or simply celebrating that it's Friday, have that extra glass of wine and eat some french fries. Leaving the door cracked lets you decide when to indulge a bit and when to hold back. It puts *you* in the driver's seat, not the food in front of you.

It's funny, but when you cook a meal, you relish in your food a little more than you would otherwise. You stay conscious of tasting every bite because you want to experience this wonderful creation of yours. You notice the flavors, and you consider how the ingredients are nourishing your body. As much as you can, cook. Cooking also tends to be healthier simply because you are using raw foods that are close to their natural source. When I cook, I start nearly every meal with

---

[11] *AARP: The Magazine*, "Eating Disorders and Women over 50," accessed April 22, 2022, https://www.aarp.org/health/conditions-treatments/info-08-2013/midlife-eating-disorders.html.

a splash of olive oil and garlic in the pan. You can wait on the garlic until the last minute before throwing in your meat and veggies so you don't burn it, but this combination of flavors is at the core of many of my meals. From there, spices determine which direction it takes.

Of course, you can't cook every day. Let's be real. Sometimes you go through the drive-through. The other day we were road tripping and we had gone through all the healthy snacks I had packed beforehand, and we were hungry—I mean, who's going to pack an egg-salad sandwich on whole wheat? Maybe you do, and if so, I take my hat off to you. But we were hungry, and we stopped at Wendy's, and I had a fish-fillet sandwich. Yeah, it's fried, and that's not great, but I ate just a few fries and handed the rest to my husband, Otto. When fast food is the rare exception, not the rule, you are doing just fine.

Here's something else. You need to determine your ideal weight rather than letting some outside source dictate what it should be. I followed a certain weight-loss program, and they suggested I aim for a very low number, which I knew I would never hit. I failed before I even got started! They determined the number by my height, but they didn't take into account that there are different body types. Some people have small bones, some big. Some people are really muscular, others petite. I've landed on an ideal weight for me, which keeps me feeling fit and looking good without sending me into stress mode around eating (after, of course, burning that unrealistic and dehumanizing number out of my brain). Find your own happy zone with your weight. Remember, it can be a gentle range rather than one harsh number.

When you step on the scale and weigh your body, make sure to weigh yourself just against yourself—no one else—and also put on the scale everything you are grateful for in your life to balance out any self-judgment that might bubble up. The numbers on the scale don't tell you how happy you are from trying a new yoga pose or why your skin is glowing after a walk or how satisfied you feel after a great time with a friend. They don't tell you how much energy you have or if you are weak from a lack of calories. Keep your eye on the full picture of happiness.

> **When you step on the scale, weigh it all, including everything that you're grateful for.**

Maybe you lost a few pounds and you are on top of the rainbow, so you think, "I'm going to keep this up, I'm going to starve myself until I am thinner than I ever imagined." What happens if you don't meet that strict (and likely unrealistic) goal? We have to accept that in our fifties, our metabolism slows down, and our lifestyle becomes a bit more sedentary. It doesn't have to be that way, but in general, it's true. And it's natural to adjust our expectations. We don't have to match the weight of what we looked like in a favorite photo from twenty years ago. Let's make a pact to be more forgiving with ourselves. You might not look like you did when you were thirty, but you can still look and feel fantastic.

Make peace with the scale. I used to imagine a happy face or sad face on the scale, depending on the number. When I got that way, I'd look at myself in the mirror and ask, "Who are you doing this for?" It was a good reminder to do it for me and not others. You control the scale; it doesn't control you. Every woman is different. Some weigh themselves several times a day; some limit themselves to once a day; others opt for once a week. Some throw the scale away and measure how well they are maintaining their weight by how their clothes fit instead. There is no right answer. Find what works for you.

When the number on the scale makes me want to dive under the covers, I remind myself that weight shifts with water retention or with muscle gain. I've read that weight can fluctuate as much as five to six pounds a day! It depends on what you eat, how much water you drink, how much salt you put on your food, whether or not you are active, and even how well you sleep. I remind myself to be patient with myself.

I have often wished that I appreciated my young, healthy, fit, and flexible body when I was young instead of worrying that it wasn't perfect. Now that I'm older, I realize how beautiful I actually was. I have turned that regret into motivation to love my body now, just as it is. I respect it by enhancing its beauty, but I have let go of the body shame that haunted me in the past.

Journaling has been a powerful tool that I have used throughout my life. It has helped me in practical ways, like keeping track of my weekly exercise and the healthy food I've eaten each day (which I personally find motivating—it's like giving myself credit). Yet it is also a place where I work through my feelings, look my challenges in the eye, and map a way to joy and peace. In chapter 5, we'll dive into the power of journaling as a tool for keeping us on track with our healthy goals and as a journey to self-love. With each day that passes, we are stronger.

HERO POSE

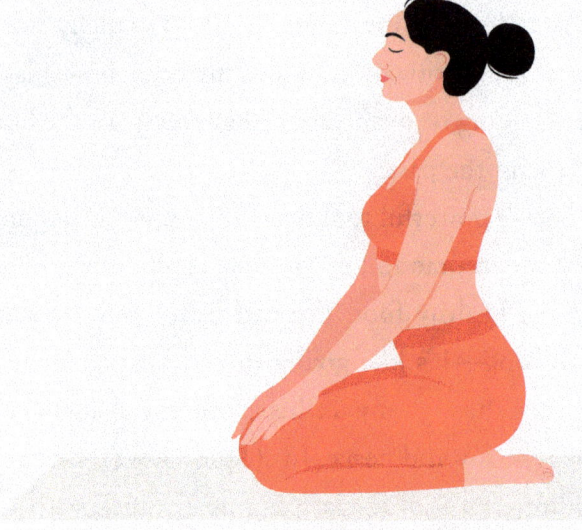

MOVE WITH MEANING

You've done some hard work with your downward dog; now it's time to sit back, reflect, and stretch your thigh muscles in hero pose. Hero pose is a bit of a break before you move forward, allowing yourself to appreciate your body and its abilities. Note: If you have knee issues, skip this pose and opt for a comfortable sitting position.

1. Come down to a kneeling position on the floor and sit back.
2. Touch your knees together, allowing your feet to rest in a somewhat wide stance behind you.
3. Lean your body slightly forward and place your hands on your upper thighs above your knees.
4. Feel the stretch in your thighs, which are pressed to the floor.
5. Like the proud warrioress that you are, lengthen your tailbone, push your shoulder blades back, and lift your sternum.

Spend about a minute in hero pose, or as long as you can. For an extra stretch, lie back into reclining hero pose with your arms reaching over your head. Think about a hardship you recently overcame and the skills you brought to the table to address it. Consider the healthy ways you take care of your body. Before rising, pat yourself on your back for being the wise, wonderful woman that you are.

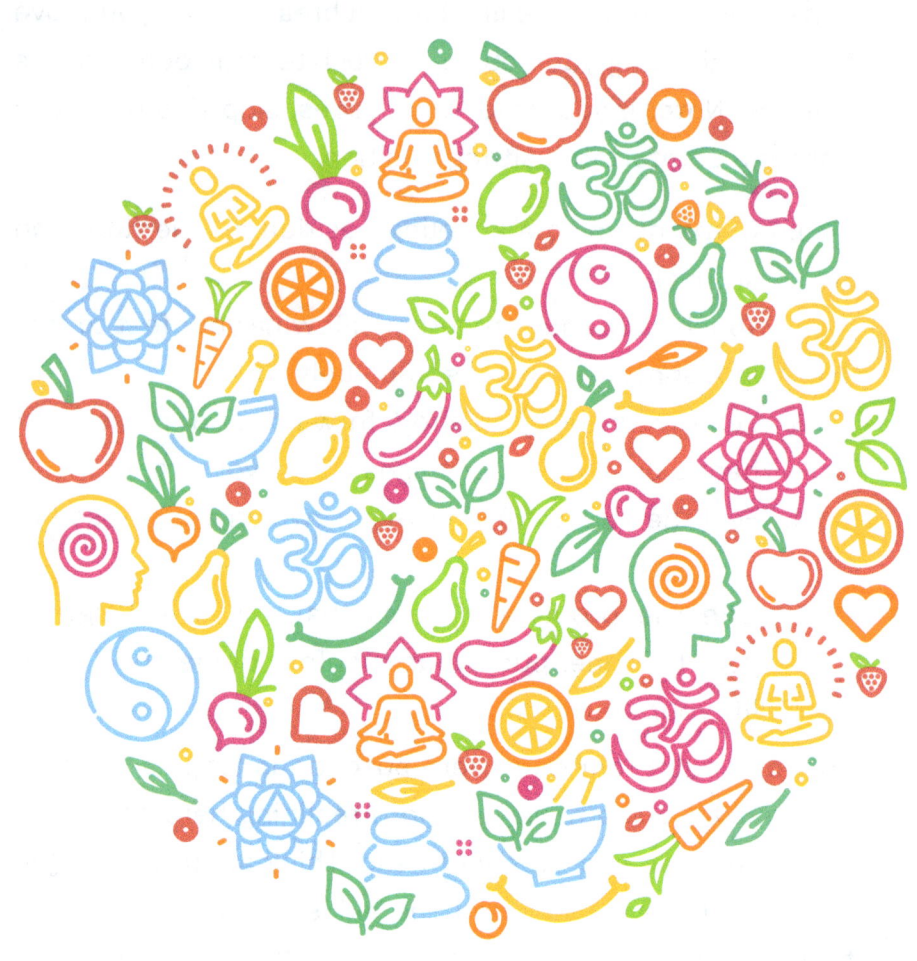

CHAPTER 5

Journal Your Way to Happiness

Settle into the Satisfaction of Sunday Dinner

Dinners at my house growing up were usually five-course affairs. They would start with antipasti and end with Italian cheesecake or another kind of Italian delicacy that could only be found at our neighborhood deli. I loved going to the deli with my mother. I can still smell the aroma of those big, fresh wheels of Parmesan.

Sundays in an Italian household means Sunday pasta. You probably refer to the topping as "sauce." Well, not us Italians. To us, it's "gravy." Gravy for Italians is a tomato sauce with meat, like Bolognese, ground beef, or sausage. Sunday dinner has been etched into my very being ever since I can remember. Even when our nest is empty, Otto and I make Sunday dinner for just us two. There's always red wine (at least for me) at the start and dessert and espresso at the end.

On holidays, Sunday pasta becomes full-blown Sunday dinner. We start with antipasti, and the Sunday pasta is served with a vegetable side, salad, dessert, and of course bread. Planning for Sunday dinner often requires a trip to the bakery to get authentic Italian bread, which is wider and rounder than French bread and, in my humble, unbiased opinion, tastier. To do it right, you have to serve it with olive oil on the side for dipping. Yum! Sure, Sunday dinner adds up to two heavy starches in one meal, but it also adds up to double the love. When you grow up in an Italian household, food is equated with love. It's a beautiful thing for sure, but it's probably a good thing that Sunday dinner is just for holidays or special family gatherings. One of my favorite vegetable side dishes is my mom's simple broccoli with lemon sauce. It's not a customary Italian dish, but she was health conscious, and it helps to balance out the pasta.

Another way I balance my life and daily diet is by keeping a log in my journal about what I eat and how much I moved my body. I don't do it every day. (I'm not perfect. Far from it. In fact, I believe that "perfection" is a four-letter word!) Yet when I do journal, I always feel more centered. It helps me make sense of my sometimes chaotic, hectic life. So does spending time laughing and talking with my family over Sunday pasta, which we of course call Sunday Gravy, and Salad Extraordinaire.

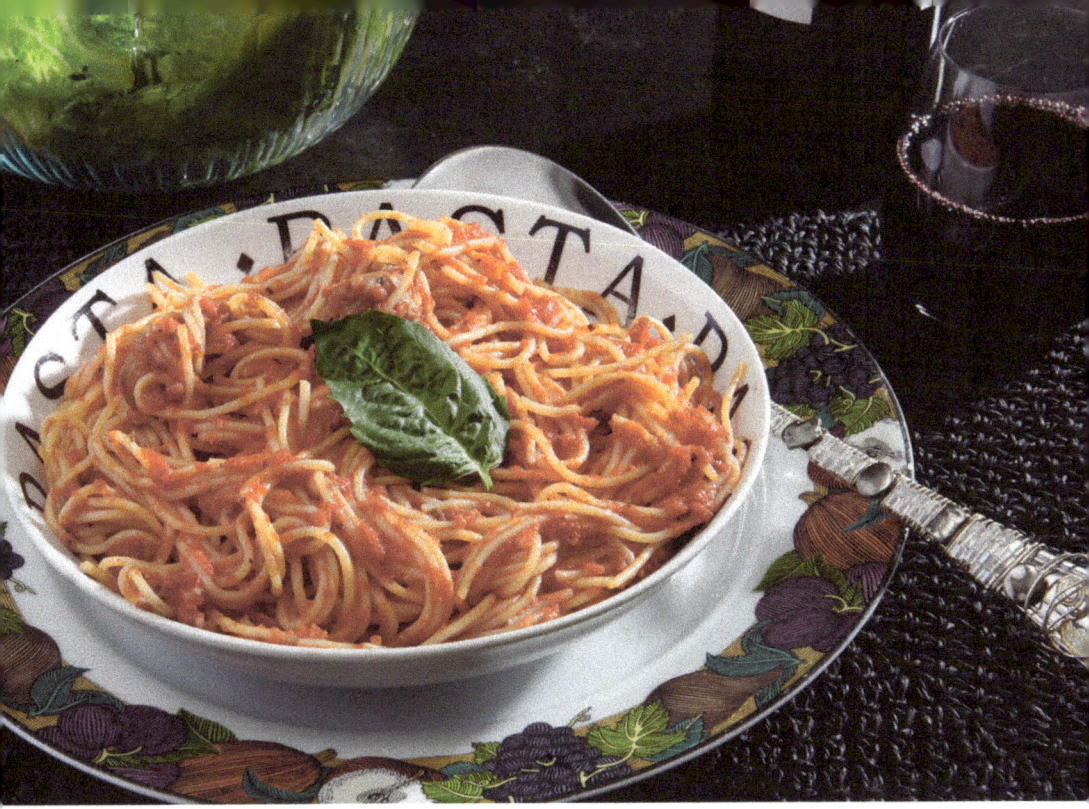

Sunday Gravy & Salad Extraordinaire

Sunday Gravy

3 teaspoons olive oil

2 cloves garlic, thinly sliced

1 teaspoon oregano

2 cans pureed tomatoes

1 pound pork sausage and/or ground beef

1 pound pasta (try linguini or farfalle, also called bow tie)

Salt and pepper to taste

Prepare sauce first: sauté garlic in oil, over medium heat, without burning! Brown meat. Add tomatoes, salt, pepper, and oregano and combine well. Keep sauce cooking over low heat for at least 30 minutes, stirring often. Prepare pasta while sauce simmers. Mix together and serve.

Salad Extraordinaire

1 head romaine lettuce, chopped

1 cucumber, thickly sliced

½ cup cherry tomatoes

2 teaspoons olive oil

1 teaspoon balsamic vinegar

Salt and pepper, to taste

Toss and enjoy!

If it's a special occasion, don't forget the bread dipped in olive oil! It's too satisfying to pass up. And if you feel like baking, add in my Pizza Dulce Cheesecake, featured in chapter 6. It's delicious, just like journaling. Journaling is like having an intimate conversation with yourself and savoring every bite. It's just you talking with yourself, so it's easy to have a real conversation and share your thoughts or feelings honestly. Or you can simply use your journal to check in with yourself on what you ate that day.

Come to think of it, maybe trusting my journal throughout my life instead of a past friend or two could've been smart! Journaling affirms your relationship with yourself and your relationship with food. I didn't journal when I was young, and I wish I would have. But it's never too late to start.

QUAINT CHILDHOOD PASTIME OR POWERFUL TOOL FOR TRANSFORMATION?

Maybe you kept a journal as a young child. Looking back, you might think it was a sweet or even frivolous pursuit, but journaling has real benefits, no matter your age. Today, you don't need a little flower-covered book with a lock and key; you can just get on your computer, tablet, or cell phone and start typing. Before you say you are too busy to journal, consider this. According to WebMD, the simple practice of writing down thoughts and feelings can reduce stress, help you gain valuable insight, spark creative problem-solving, and allow you to see situations in a new light. It's not only good for your mental health but your physical health too. Researchers found that people with medical conditions and anxiety who journaled fifteen minutes for three days a week over a twelve-week period increased feelings of well-being and had fewer depressive symptoms.[12] So before you write off journaling, give it a try. You just might find you are calmer and better at handling what life throws your way, and we all need more of that!

---

12   WebMD, "Mental Health Benefits of Journaling," accessed June 7, 2022, https://www.webmd.com/mental-health/mental-health-benefits-of-journaling.

Journaling is an account of your personal history, and reading through past journals can provide valuable insight into your personal growth. It helps you laugh at the times when you felt insecure or inferior when you were younger. Doesn't some of it seem so ridiculous now? How a mean comment could really set you off? Now you are wise, and you can see the meanness for what it probably was—less about you and more about the other person.

If you have journals from your past, read them to get a sense of who you were then and who you are now. Celebrate your growth and also recognize that young spirit that's still in you, wanting to take on the world. Embrace your wisdom. You've learned a lot about yourself, life, and others, so you can trust yourself. Trust feels like the satisfaction after a fun weekend when you sit down to eat some pasta with a healthy twist for Sunday dinner.

Feelings are a part of life. If you are feeling sad, worried, or anxious, dig deep and muck around in the source of your feelings while you get them out on paper. There's a good chance you will see a solution in the end or gain a new perspective. I see it as taking out the garbage. By removing the crud, you make room for fresh thoughts and feelings to flow in.

When you become aware of what you are feeling, it's sheer power. You can make choices about what works and what doesn't work in your life. You can set healthy boundaries with other people. You can spend time doing the things that bring you the most joy. When you become aware of the source of your thoughts and feelings, you are better able to choose to do something to improve your mood. With self-awareness, you become more present. To live our best lives as women in our fifties, we have to try to be more vulnerable—even when it rearranges the furniture of our lives.

To age gracefully, truly gracefully, we have to face our feelings that are right under the rug.

Some people swear by a gratitude journal (and so do their therapists)! If you are not sleeping well, try journaling a few minutes before bed about what you are grateful for in your life. It helps you fall asleep because you are not focused on what you didn't get done that day or a negative interaction that happened. You are looking at what is working in your life, not what's going wrong. You are counting your wins, not your failures. That alone makes you feel better about yourself and happier with your life.

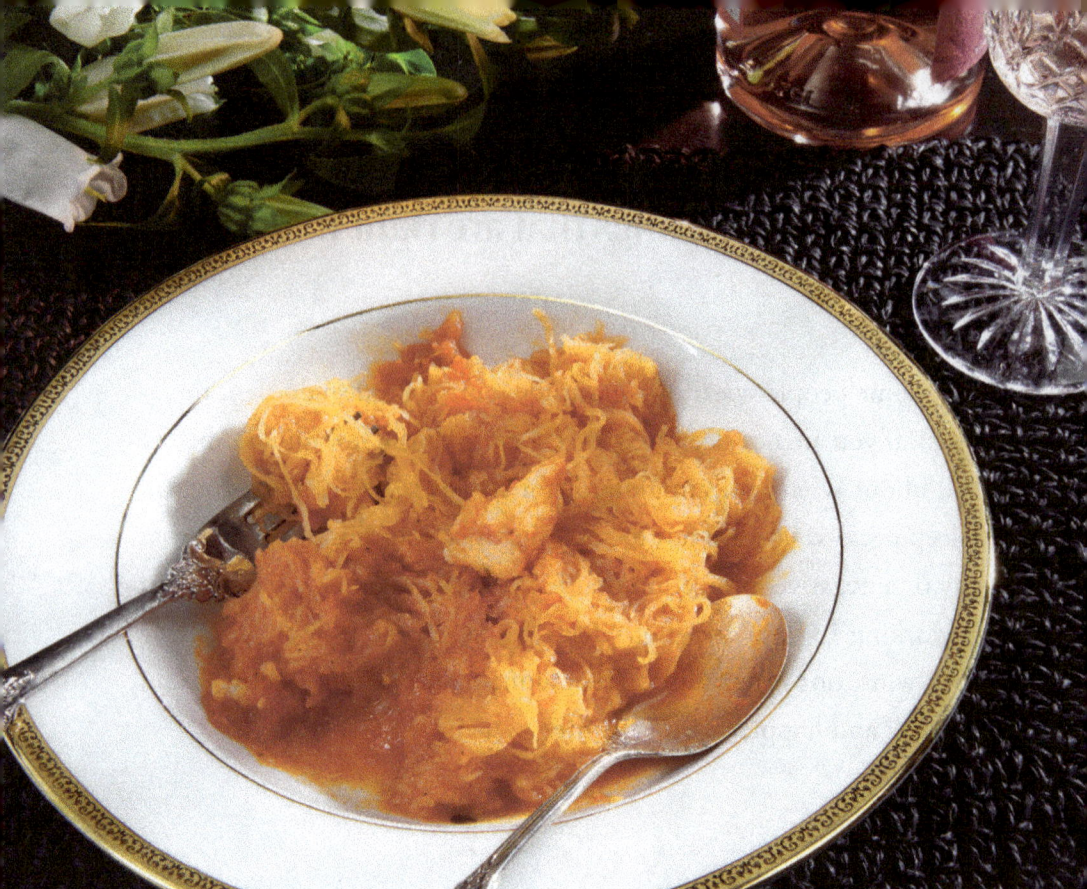

Spaghetti Squash Marinara with Scallops or Shrimp

- 1 spaghetti squash
- 1 cup scallops or shrimp, fresh or defrosted
- 2 cups marinara sauce

Marinara (the Italian answer to everything!):

- 3 cans chopped tomatoes
- ½ cup extra-virgin olive oil
- 2 cloves garlic, thinly sliced
- 1 teaspoon oregano
- Salt and pepper to taste

Prepare the marinara by adding garlic to olive oil and simmering for about a minute over medium heat. Add tomato, oregano, salt, and pepper. Bring to boil. Cover and simmer on low heat for 30 to 40 minutes. While marinara simmers, parboil the squash (boil in salted water for 5 minutes). Slice in half and remove seeds, then bake on baking tray at 350°F for 20 minutes. Scrape squash into strings. Sauté the scallops or shrimp in a little olive oil in a saucepan for 4 to 5 minutes. Pour the marinara sauce over squash. Mix in the seafood. Voilà!

Create a ritual around journaling. Find a quiet place, sip a favorite drink, and dream a little. If I'm making plans or creating lists, I drink coffee. It perks me up and gives me confidence. But if I'm contemplating my feelings, I sip tea. For me, a steaming cup of chamomile tea instantly relaxes me. It takes away my anxiety, and my brain just floats.

Making journaling a ritual helps me tap into my philosophical side, where I contemplate life and enjoy inspiring mantras that pop into my mind. I pretty much come up with a new one every day! Mantras are good for the soul. When I need to release some anxiety, I repeat to myself, "I feel confident and clear headed" quietly while sitting and sipping tea, and it works. It's a perfect setup for journaling.

FEELING BRAVE? JOURNAL ABOUT WHAT'S HOLDING YOU BACK

Some of our thought patterns and beliefs can hold us back (and they need to go in the trash)! Grab your journal or notebook and spend a few moments journaling about each one of the prompts below. Remember, your opinion of yourself is the only one that matters! You've gained strength and wisdom through the years, and now you can let go of negative self-messaging and step into your future with confidence.

- If you could turn back the clock, what would you do differently? Is there something you regret? Every single person has some regrets. How can you change that decision or action, today, so that you can release it?
- How did people define you when you were young? Name five ways your friends or family described you in your teen years. Which of these characteristics still ring true today? If a certain way of being doesn't resonate with you, acknowledge it and release it, as in "I am no longer afraid to try new things."
- What beliefs do you carry about yourself from when you were young that no longer serve you? For example, "I'm not athletic," "I'm shy," "I'm too loud," "I don't have interesting things to say." Examine where these beliefs originated. If they

feel false, what small steps can you take to prove them wrong moving forward?
- What is a passion that you never pursued? Is there a hidden talent that needs attention? How can you start taking baby steps toward it today?

Hiding our feelings or pushing down our desires never works. Commit to journaling, even if it's just now and then when you are in the mood. When I journal, I become aware of what I want more of in life. I can see where I'm wasting my energy and what I would rather be doing instead. Everyone needs improvement. We are not perfect beings, and that's okay, so what do you want to improve upon? If you feel nervous or anxious about something, meditate or journal about it. Being honest with ourselves helps us know ourselves better, and that knowing leads to confidence from the inside out.

Let's say you want to start a plan to move every day to improve your health. I say just start. Don't judge yourself about how out of shape you are. You can only improve from where you are if that's what you want! If you are not used to moving, walk around the block regularly for a week. The next week, add another loop. Make it a part of your plan to improve your life. It will build on itself, and before you know it, you will be improving your life in other ways too.

How about making exercise fun by inviting friends to join you? Now and then I have yoga parties where my crazy group of friends comes over for a free yoga class, provided by me, and a social hour afterward. Sometimes we enjoy a glass of wine along with my favorite Prosciutto Banana Pepper Pizza, which I cut into strips and present as an appetizer.

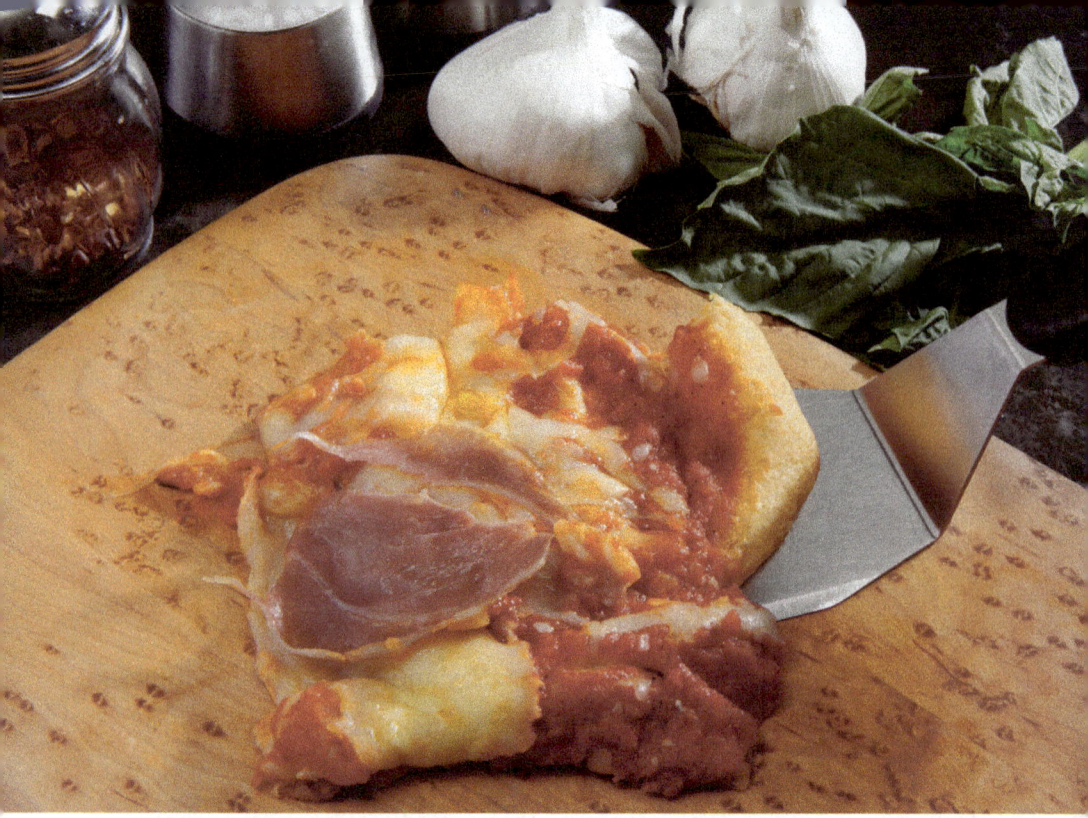

Prosciutto Banana Pepper Pizza

1 crust (from store for ease)
¼ cup marinated banana peppers
1½ cups shredded mozzarella cheese
1 cup prepared marinara sauce (or make it from scratch—see the previous recipe)
2 large slices prosciutto Italian ham
¼ cup olive oil

Brush crust with oil. Spread sauce, add cheese, and then add ham and peppers. Bake at 425°F for 12 minutes. It's so good I sometimes eat it for breakfast!

If you are gaining weight and you want to see where extra calories are sneaking in, you might try journaling what you eat every day for a week. In the past, I would go on these crazy crash diets and lose perspective. Italian women tend to be voluptuous and often short, not what the "ideal" female body was supposed to look like in the '80s and '90s. Things got confusing there for a while as I tried to meld reality with fantasy.

When I explored crash dieting in my journal, I recognized that I wasn't thinking clearly in the past. Journaling helped me see that I didn't need to diet to maintain my weight. I didn't need to obsess over every calorie I ate. Instead, I could focus on healthy food that fed my body and fed my happiness. (And if I wanted to lose a pound or two, I could loosely count my calories and be gentle with myself along the way.) Today, instead of going on an extreme diet, I simply put up a few easy guideposts for eating and exercise and happily live my life in between them, making food my friend, not my foe.

The goal of a food journal is not to figure out how to starve yourself. Not at all. It's to recognize patterns. Do you eat more when you skip a snack? Do you do better with protein for breakfast? What time during the day do you naturally get hungry for dinner? Do you eat when you are lonely? It's all information to put the power in your hands when it comes to maintaining a healthy weight for you.

Journaling is living life with your eyes wide open. From journaling, I learned that if I skip meals, I overeat. I also learned that I would gain weight during stressful times because I ate to comfort myself—to soothe my feelings or reward myself after a long day—rather than a way to nourish my body.

Here's a sample entry from my food journal. You will see that I include not just what I eat but how much activity I get in a day. As you learned in chapter 1, I'm dedicated to eating five times a day and sometimes a dessert.

MARIA'S SAMPLE FOOD JOURNAL ENTRY

Date: Oct. 5, 2021

Weight: Lost 2 lbs. this month

Activity: Walk 1 mile; housework; walk the dog

Breakfast: Applesauce/coffee with collagen peptides

Snack: 5 rice cakes

Lunch: Chicken with broccoli

Snack: 1 cup popcorn

Dinner: Brown rice noodles with broccoli and tofu, one glass of red wine

Dessert: Baked apple with dollop of whipped cream

Feelings: A little bloated, but happy with the day

Do me a favor and stop reading for a second to take a deep breath. Now another, with a long, slow exhale. Pat yourself on the back for being brave and taking a look at some hard stuff through journaling. When we are self-aware and move through life with intention, we tend to eat with purpose: Eating for fuel, not for comfort. Eating to share life and laughter with friends. Journaling helps us stay on track with our personal goals and tap into our passions. In the next chapter, I dive deeper into getting inspired and building a better, more satisfying life. After all, as a beautiful woman in your fifties, you deserve to live your best life, whatever you decide that might be.

JOURNAL YOUR WAY TO HAPPINESS

EAGLE POSE

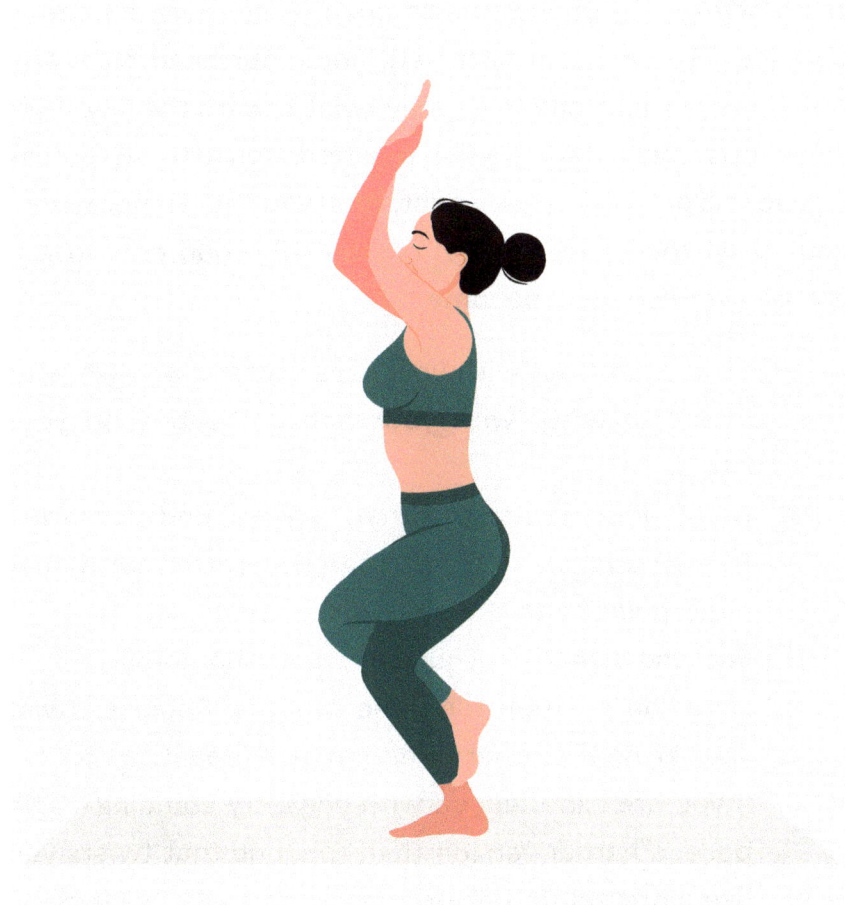

MOVE WITH MEANING

As you move out of the more contemplative hero pose, you get ready to rise up with eagle pose. Eagle pose demands balance. Tap into your core self, hold your head high, and feel power in your hands as they twist toward the sky. With eagle pose, you decide your position. You can sit cross-legged, sit on your heels, squat, or stand tall. Honor where you are in the moment. Feel regal. Feel proud of who you are and who you will become.

1. Sit on the floor with your legs crossed or with your knees together with your bottom resting on your heels.
2. Bring your arms together, palms and forearms facing, and twist them together with your upper hand pointing to the sky.
3. Feel the stretch in your arms and shoulders.
4. Hold the position for three breaths. Release. Twist your arms the other direction and repeat.
5. If you are experienced with yoga, try standing-eagle pose, a harder version than this one that twists you like a pretzel. To perform standing eagle, balance on one leg in a squatted position and twist your arms together but also twist your free leg behind your grounded leg.

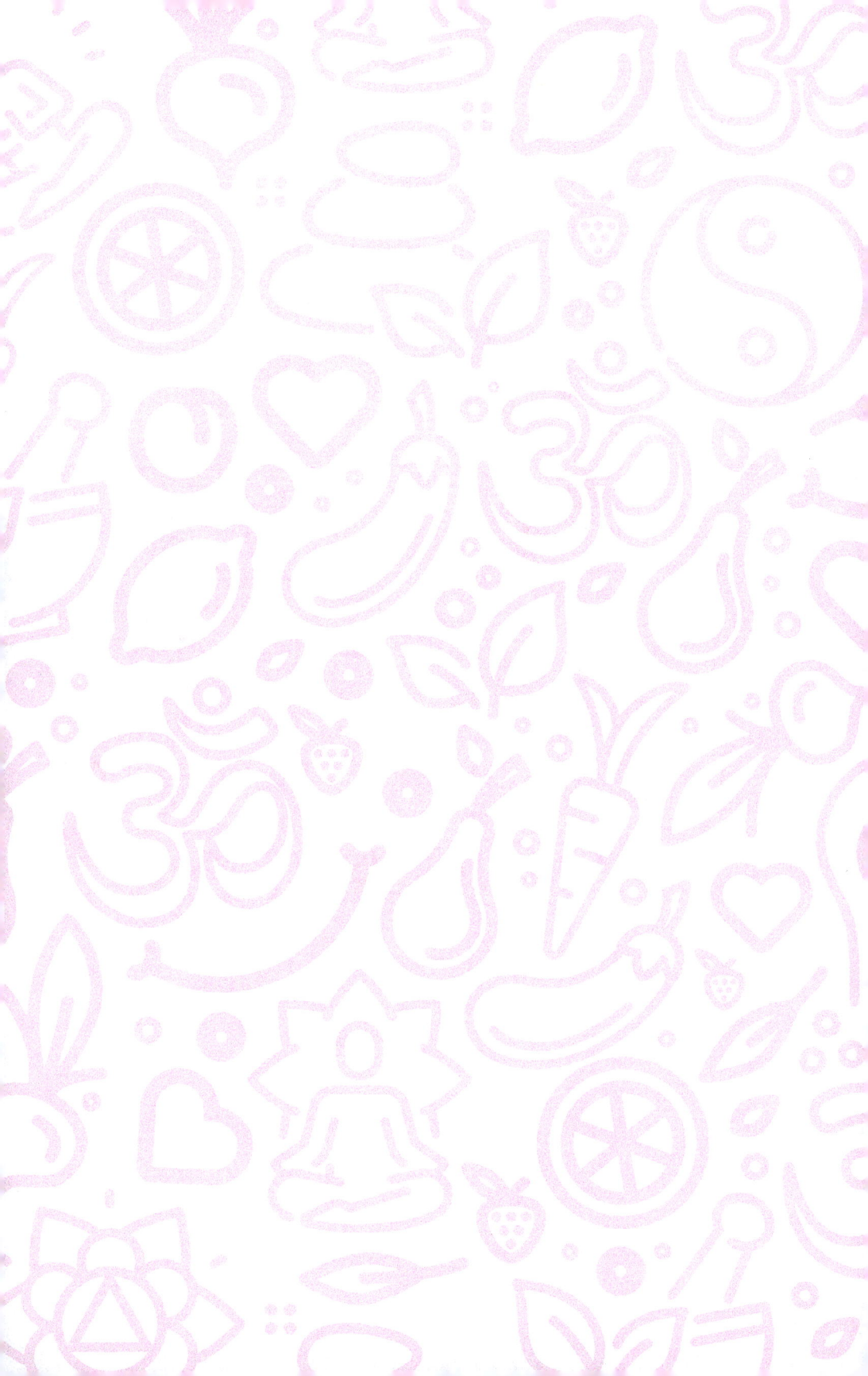

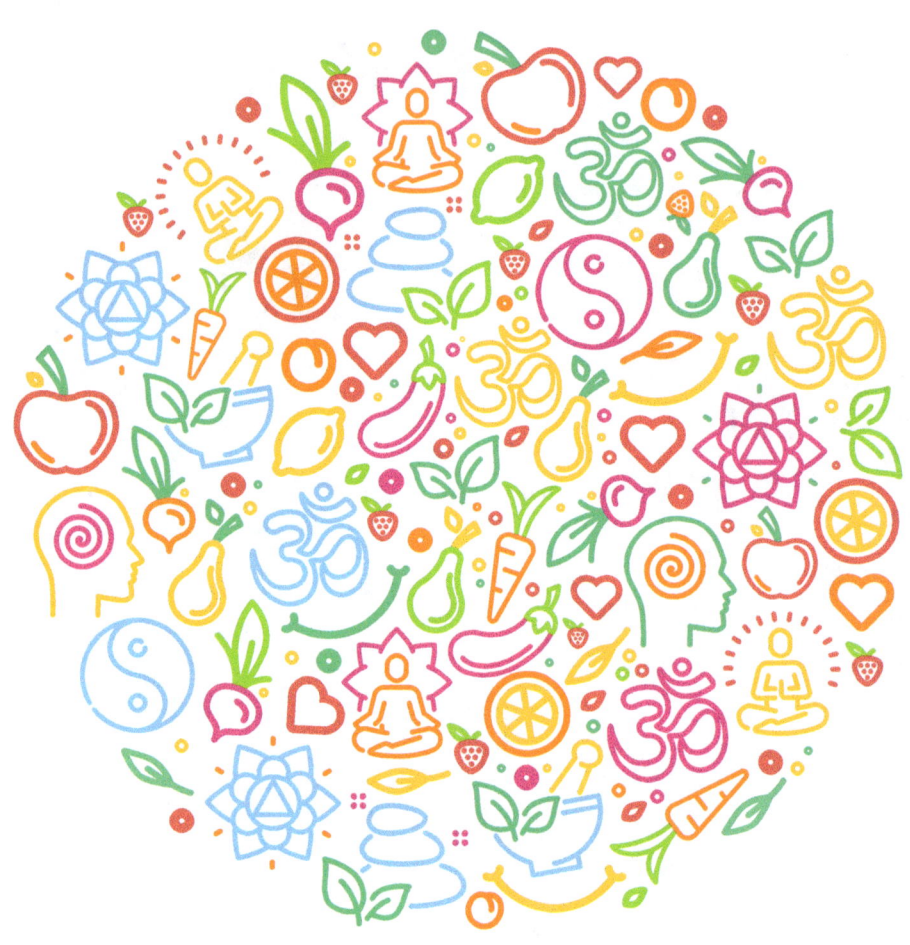

CHAPTER 6

Get Inspired!
Feel Decadent with Pizza Dulce Cheesecake

Recently, Otto and I met some old friends for dinner and dancing. The kind of friends you feel completely yourself with, like family. Toward the end of the night, a Bruce Springsteen song came on, and I'm a Jersey girl, so I couldn't contain myself. I screamed and hollered and went crazy singing and dancing along. The next morning Otto commented that I was really getting into it. He was right! It felt wonderful to cut loose. When you are singing and dancing, there's just no way you can feel bad. Plus, dancing lets the young you come out and party. Changing up your daily life with an occasional wild night out (not that we can party like we used to) is inspiring. And rich and decadent. Just like my mom's famous Pizza Dulce Cheesecake.

Pizza Dulce Cheesecake

Graham cracker crust:
2 cups graham cracker crumbs
1 stick butter, melted

Combine crumbs and melted butter. Pat in bottom and sides of a cheesecake/springform pan. Bake at 325°F for 8 to 10 minutes. Allow to cool.

Filling:
3 pounds ricotta cheese
1 cup heavy cream
1¼ cups confectioners' sugar
7 eggs
2 teaspoons orange liquor
Zest of 1 lemon
Zest of 1 orange

Beat sugar and ricotta until creamy. Add eggs, cream, liquor, and the zests and beat until well combined. Pour filling mixture into prepared crust. Bake at 375°F for 1 hour, until filling is firm and center is a little wobbly. Turn off the oven; leave cake in the oven with the door partially opened for 30 minutes. Refrigerate when cool.

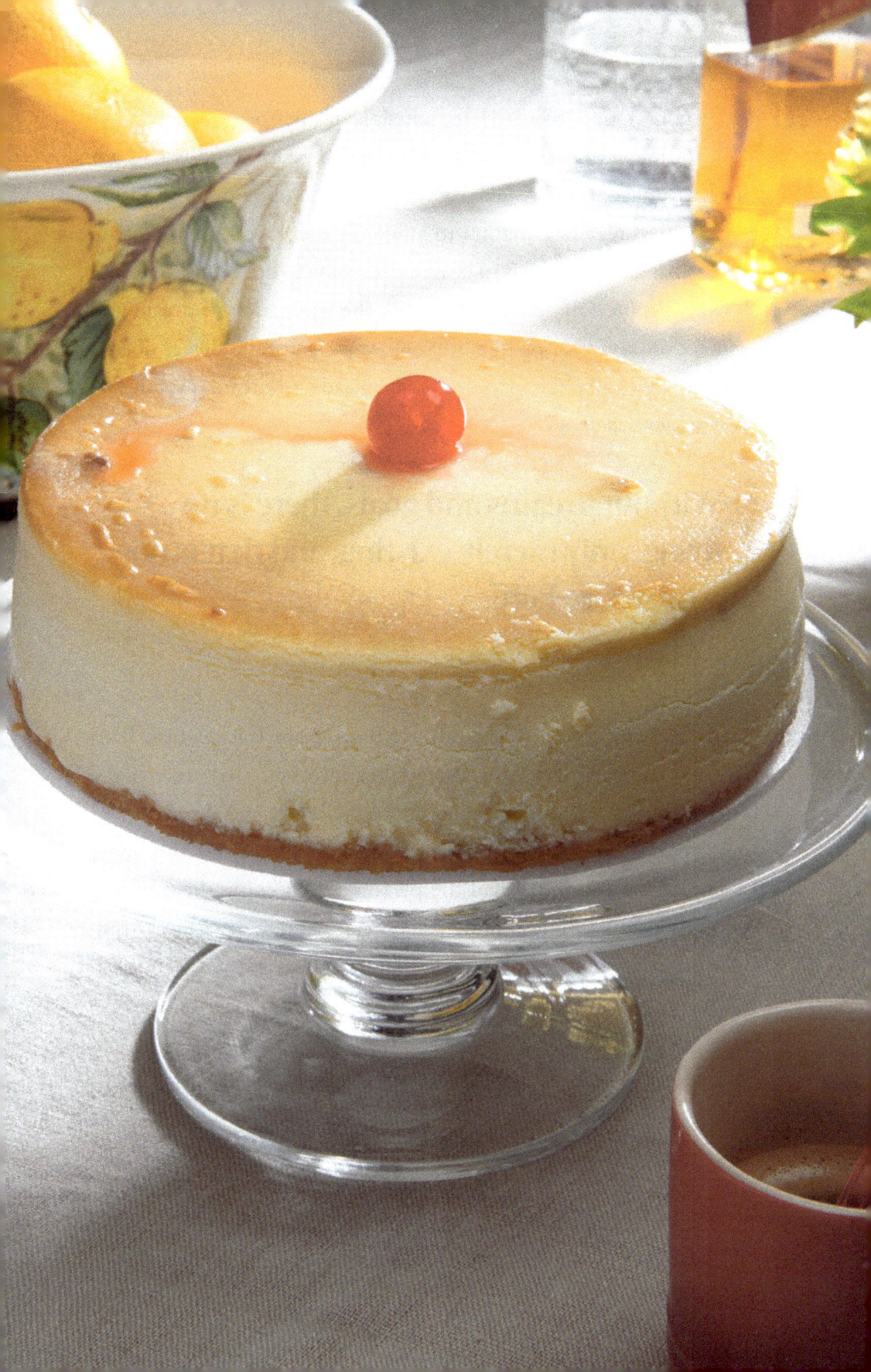

You may have noticed that I am a major idea person. Picture a caricature of me with a giant light bulb above my head, and you've got the right image. It seems like every day I come up with an inspiring new business idea or a mantra to guide my life. With me, there's no holding back. My nature is to be an extremist who doesn't do anything halfway. I appreciate this about myself, the willingness to dream and then act on my dreams. Just because we are getting older, it doesn't mean that we can't have dreams! So go ahead and dream, even if you don't achieve them all.

> **Without dreams and goals, there is no living, only merely existing, and that is not why we are here.**
> —Mark Twain

I have something that I call my Big Dream Bucket List. It's a mash-up of goals that seem attainable and others that seem like a big stretch, but hey, becoming aware of my hopes and dreams is the first step in making them come true! In fact, while writing this book, I completed a few, and I had the pleasure of checking them off my list. After reading mine, I hope you go crazy and make a Big Dream Bucket List of your own. Remember, it's a bucket list, not a guilt list. It is for inspiration, not accountability.

MARIA'S BIG DREAM BUCKET LIST

- ✓ Write a book
- ✓ Eat delicious food in Italy
- ○ Tour the Grand Canyon with my family
- ○ Renew my wedding vows with my husband in Las Vegas
- ○ Go on safari in South Africa
- ○ Start my own line of makeup
- ○ Have my own cooking show
- ○ Have a combo dance/yoga/spirituality studio
- ○ Open a takeout restaurant called Maria's Miracle Salads
- ○ Start a makeup-training business called Maria's Makeovers, which I'd run out of my own salon and where I'm the lead makeup artist
- ○ Earn a million dollars

Dreaming takes away all limits and blows the doors wide open. Anything is possible. Dreaming is pure inspiration that leads to real change through goal setting. As a mother of two teenagers who are now both off to college, I find that having a bucket list helps ease the empty-nest syndrome. If you are a mother, it's a major transition when your kids leave home. You pour everything you've got into your kids, and then suddenly, poof, they are out on their own and you find yourself with time on your hands. Try not to wallow; instead, see all your extra time as an opportunity. It's the perfect time to dedicate yourself to your own dreams and goals.

It's also a great time to get back to doing something you loved to do when you were young. Like I said earlier, I love to dance. When I was young, I did ballet and even performed as a child in the New Jersey Ballet. In my late twenties, I had the privilege of taking a jazz class that was taught by a dancer who played one of the Sharks in *West Side Story*. It's one of my small claims to fame! In reality, it was a jazz class that was open to everybody, but it lit a fire in me.

I'm now coming full circle. I signed up for an adult jazz class at the dance school that my daughters used to attend. Being older, it feels gutsy to put myself out there. I tease my daughters that it is payback time—I have attended more dance recitals through the years than I can count, and now they have to come to mine! It feels good to be stepping out of my comfort zone and challenging myself in this way. It's a goal that I get to check off of a mini bucket list.

What goals do you have that are a running theme in your life? What did you enjoy as a teenager that you could pick up again? Passions often stick with us; they just need a lit match to get them burning again.

Goals are dreams broken into small steps. Goals are grounded in everyday life. Personally, while I like to create dream bucket lists, I'm not so hot on goal lists. (I said I was an idea person!) With goals, I tend to be more casual. I bite off my goals in small pieces and I keep them in mind as suggestions more than a rule book for life. I take a kinder, gentler approach to goal setting than some people, but we all have to honor who we are and what works for us. What's your style when it comes to dreaming or setting goals?

I've learned as a wise, older, exciting woman that once I put a goal in writing, it becomes real. That can be a great thing for keeping me on track, or it can backfire and make me feel bad about myself. I often say the first rule of life should be "Don't make yourself crazy!"

If you are like me, and writing down goals and checking them off isn't your style, you could try choosing one goal at a time and concentrating on that. Maybe it's simply quitting work at a reasonable hour so you can exercise before dinner. Do it until it's a habit; then work on the next goal. I've learned that if I go slow and steady with positive goals, they add up fast.

SET A GOAL TO SET SOME GOALS

Have you been thinking that you need to set some goals, but you haven't found the time to do so? That intention is a goal in and of itself! The idea of goal setting can feel overwhelming, but setting goals can ultimately increase your satisfaction by helping you feel more focused, more productive, and more efficient.[13] When setting goals, remember the four Cs:

1. **Commitment.** Without commitment, the whole process loses its purpose. Within your goal is a promise to yourself—a contract of sorts—that will spur you on to achieving your goal.
2. **Clarity.** Be clear and specific when setting goals. A vague goal without specifics for achieving it will be more likely to fall off your radar. Rather than saying, "I'm going to join a gym," say, "I'm going to visit four gyms by the end of the month and sign up within a week of choosing one."

---

13 Positive Psychology, "What Is Goal Setting and How to Do It Well," accessed June 9, 2022, https://positivepsychology.com/goal-setting/.

3. **Challenging.** Achieving harder goals builds your confidence, gives you that sense of control, and adds meaning to your life.
4. **Complexity.** While you might want to climb Mount Everest, that's not going to happen immediately. Choose a doable goal, like joining a climbing gym or taking a climbing class to start. Set your sights high but be realistic. After all, attaining your goal is the ultimate goal!

One of my goals through the years has been to run a marathon within my lifetime. I haven't done it yet, but it doesn't mean I have given up on it! When I see a marathoner who is in their eighties crossing the finish line, I think they must have special powers. More likely, it's persistence, dedication, and a crazy inner drive. I am always curious about what motivates older runners to push through the aches and pains and stay so active and healthy.

I don't jog as much as I used to, but I still do once in a while. The other day I took a different route than I usually do. I discovered that seeing new sights and hearing new sounds was really refreshing to me. It's so important to avoid falling into a rut, which is an easy thing to do when our lives are settled in our fifties. Join me in doing something new to shake things up, even if it's just taking a different route when walking or running, or trying a new exercise class at the gym. I also suggest trying a new healthy yet tasty recipe, like my Baked Apple.

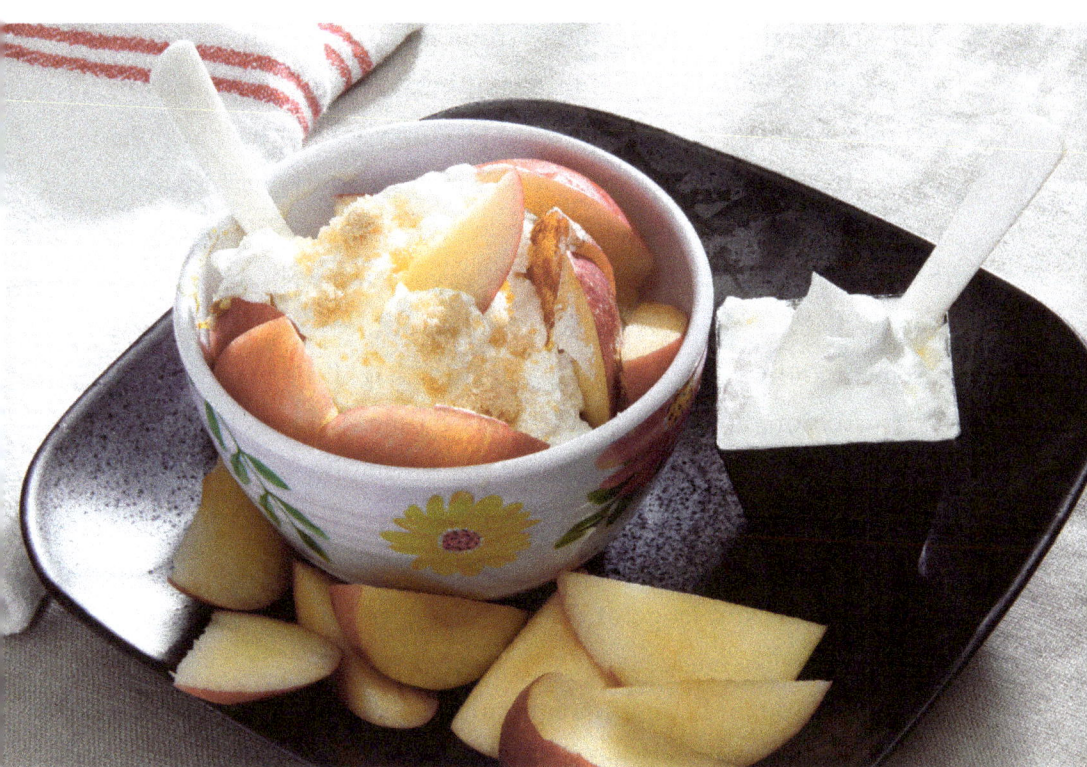

Baked Apple

- 1 apple, quartered
- ½ cup water
- 1 teaspoon cinnamon
- 1 teaspoon sugar
- ¼ cup whipped cream or nondairy topping

Put the apple in a bowl of water. Steam it in the microwave for a few minutes until soft. Drain the water and top with remaining ingredients.

Motivation is the wheel that moves inspiration forward. It transports an idea out of your head and into your life. Let's take exercise as an example. Maybe you are inspired to take up yoga but haven't done it yet. Here's a tip to get you going: time your workout with your moods. When you feel anxious, stressed, or agitated, do something that demands a burst of energy. Besides yoga and walking, another exercise I do is kickboxing. When I feel all pent up, I go to the basement and take it out on my punching bag. It's great! I get out my frustration, and I get fit at the same time. I always feel better afterward, when both my body and my frustration are spent. Find your punching bag. Something that lets you get negativity out and makes you feel strong. Something that lets you forget about your responsibilities and let go of the day. Being stressed gets in the way of inspiration, so release it.

Inspiration and commitment go hand in hand. One offers the get up and go, and the other the ability to stick to it. If you find it hard to get inspired, maybe you need someone else to motivate you. I used to work with a personal trainer, which really helped me stay committed to my workout routine. His motivation rubbed off on me and inspired me to keep going. Being accountable to someone works magic. If you are having trouble fitting enough movement and exercise into your week, try setting up a weekly walk with a friend or finding a gym buddy who will meet you a few times a week.

When you are committed to living healthily—eating nourishing foods and staying active—you will be amazed by how it opens you up to creativity and inspiration in other areas of your life. Having set commitments and routines keeps us on track for reaching our goals and dreams. Add in persistence and patience, and you are bound to get there. But not that other *p* word, "perfection." That's a dream canceler. If we are trying to be a certain way, we are not being natural.

GET INSPIRED!

We are standing in one position, afraid to move. Perfection is like building solid walls around ourselves. Walls that do not allow us to step outside of a comfortable box. When we let go of unreachable standards for ourselves and let the walls fall, then we can start to imagine what we want in life. Let your ideas soar, even if they feel a bit silly, like how I felt when I created my delightful Berry Salad dessert with a dreamy surprise—gummy bears!

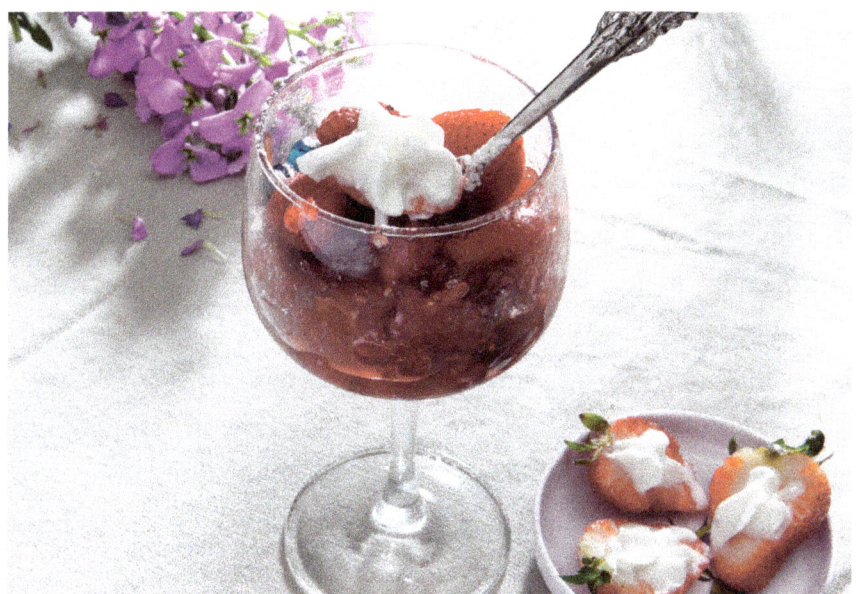

Berry Salad

- 1 mini package of gummy bears
- ½ cup chopped strawberries
- ½ cup raspberries
- 2 tablespoons confectioners' sugar or whipped cream

Mix together, sprinkle with sugar or a dab of whipped cream, and enjoy!

Feeling inspired with eating and exercise is like riding a Ferris wheel, including the satisfaction of going round and round. I gain confidence from eating well, which requires discipline and commitment. In turn, my newfound confidence spills into other areas of my life, like writing this book and creating my website on living your best life in your fifties (officialmariasabando.com). Every woman lives this cycle of inspiration, motivation, and commitment differently, but we all experience it. We all have skill and talent and drive. One success feeds into the next success and the next. Take the ride! And if you have to get off and rest now and then, that's just fine.

If you have a goal that you want to achieve but you are having a hard time knowing where to begin, consider working with a life coach. Having that extra guidance, and paying for it, is a great motivator for making change. If you don't have extra funds, rely on a trusted friend or relative who is a good listener and cheerleader. Ask if they are willing to set up a formal meeting every few weeks to talk about your goals over coffee. Remember, you don't earn an extra prize for going it alone. That old saying "If you want something done right, do it yourself" is outdated and damaging. I say ask for the help you need. In getting it, you will find your motivation.

Looking for inspiration? Get out and enjoy the arts.

Remember how I suggested shaking things up to loosen up fresh ideas? Nothing is more inspiring than witnessing other people's inspiration! Make plans to go to an art exhibit, a play, a show, a concert, or a sculpture garden. It will do you wonders to help you wake up to new possibilities, and it might even spark you to create something artistic of your own. Maybe you are already a creative, and you need motivation to do your art. Go see artists that you admire. Have you been to an art walk in your town or a town nearby? The energy artists give to the crowd and the appreciation they receive back is fun to experience.

I always wished I was a musician. I played piano for years. I know I will never sing like Barbra Streisand, but I love music. It's on my mini bucket list to pick up another instrument someday. Getting out and listening to live music feeds that inspiration for me.

What do you want to be when you grow up?

I'm just kidding—but not really. Likely, you've found your true talents, and you are deep into your career by now. But do you ever wonder where you would be today if you picked a different degree in college, or you chose to settle in a different place, or you went back to school later in life and started a new career? Our life choices have led us down a certain road, and as we grow older that road can start to become predictable. It doesn't have to be that way. It's never too late to explore a new road—a new career, business, hobby, moonlighting gig, or side hustle. Even while maintaining your regular job. Consider it with sheer pleasure, like discovering a creative new dessert like my Banana Bread Pudding.

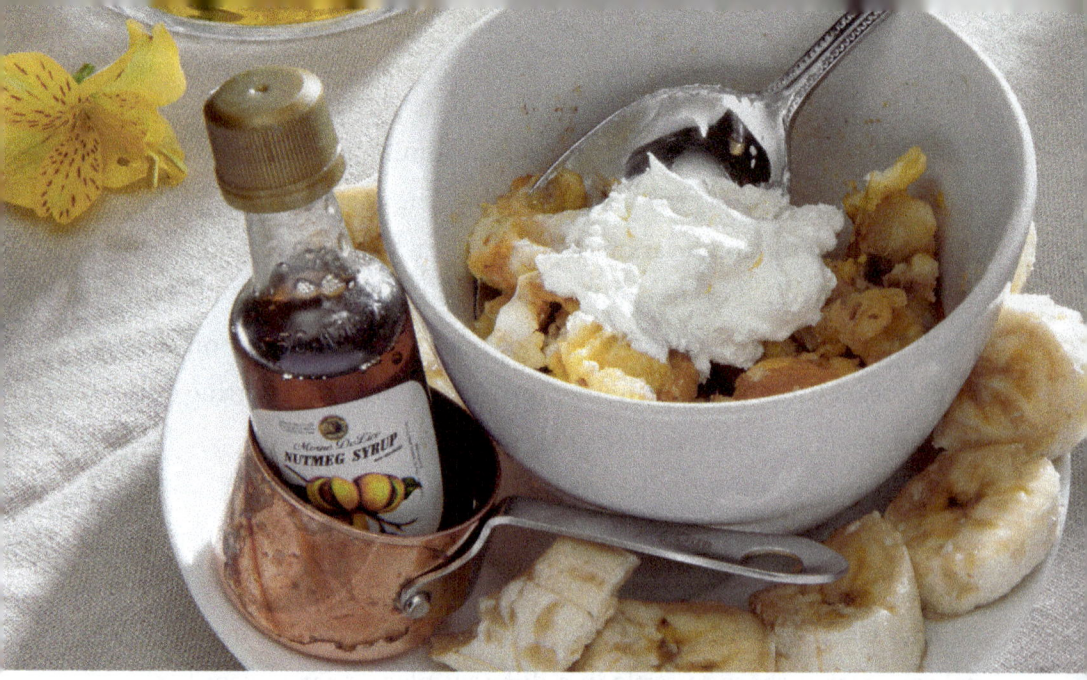

Banana Bread Pudding

- 1 banana, sliced
- 4 bakery cinnamon rolls, sliced in half
- ¼ cup milk
- 2 eggs, scrambled
- 1 teaspoon sugar
- ½ teaspoon cinnamon
- Whipped cream, dollop
- 2 teaspoons butter

Beat eggs with milk in bowl. Place roll halves in bowl with egg mixture and coat. Allow to soak for 10 minutes. Melt butter in fry pan on stove top. Fry banana slices until slightly browned, then remove from pan. Fry the soaked bread slices, flipping over a few times until browned. Layer bread and bananas in soufflé cups. Sprinkle with sugar and cinnamon and top with whipped cream.

To discover a passion that could turn into an artistic expression or a side hustle, start by meditating on activities or topics that hold your interest. What comes up? Or try thinking about who you envy or admire. Is it the woman who bakes pies and sells them at the farmers market? Or the man who paints murals in your town or city? Maybe you are inspired by beautiful photography. Pay attention to these inklings and awakenings as you go about your life. Once you identify something, learn all you can about it. Nose around on Pinterest; listen to podcasts; talk to others about your idea. Then take it for a test run by joining a class or writing out a business plan.

TIPS FOR TAPPING INTO YOUR CREATIVITY

Think you're not creative? Think again. All of us have the ability to be creative, which has a host of benefits and doesn't require that you take painting lessons—unless you want to, of course! To tap into your creative side, try the following:

- Kick your inner critic to the curb. Self-judgment puts the kibosh on flexing your creative muscles. If the critic is someone else, invite them to kindly keep their opinions to themselves. Ever notice that creativity strikes while in the shower? That's because you've made space to invite creativity in. Intentionally plan to spend time alone with no agenda to get the juices flowing.

- Hang out with like-minded people once you find your creative outlet. Choose people who can provide useful feedback, help you problem solve, or help you get unstuck if you've hit a roadblock.

- Expand your world by getting a change of scenery. Instead of hanging out at home, grab a book and spend an hour in a coffee shop. Being in a new space sparks new ideas.

- Get your body moving. An increased heart rate gets blood pumping, literally helping you to think better.[14]

You don't have to win awards and display them on your wall for your new business, hobby, or creative endeavor. You just have to feel good when you are doing it and feel like celebrating a little afterward. Also, give yourself time and space to learn and grow. I recently took up latch hook. It's like needlepoint, but it's easier. My family asks what I am going to make, but it's not about the end result; it's about enjoying the process. It's art for art's sake. Artists are often driven to create their art. It simply has to burst out of them. Give yourself permission to explore the idea that you might be a hidden artist.

> **We all have untapped talents. What's yours? Focus on your strengths and passions, and you will discover it.**

You have a ton of life experience to lend to a new venture. I hate to be so blunt, but if you are not getting busy living, you are getting busy dying, something reminiscent of what my father would say. Every year that we grow older is a gift, and getting old isn't for amateurs. If you're not thrilled about growing older, just remember that it's better than the alternative! You are still here and still alive, so savor it. Take the lessons you learned in the past and use them to live better in the future.

---

14 *Forbes*, "How to Be More Creative and Boost Happiness: 6 Ways to Get Inspired," accessed June 9, 2022, https://www.forbes.com/sites/tracy-brower/2021/07/25/how-to-be-more-creative-and-boost-happiness-6-ways-to-get-inspired/?sh=26e597857d70.

GET INSPIRED!

DANCER'S POSE

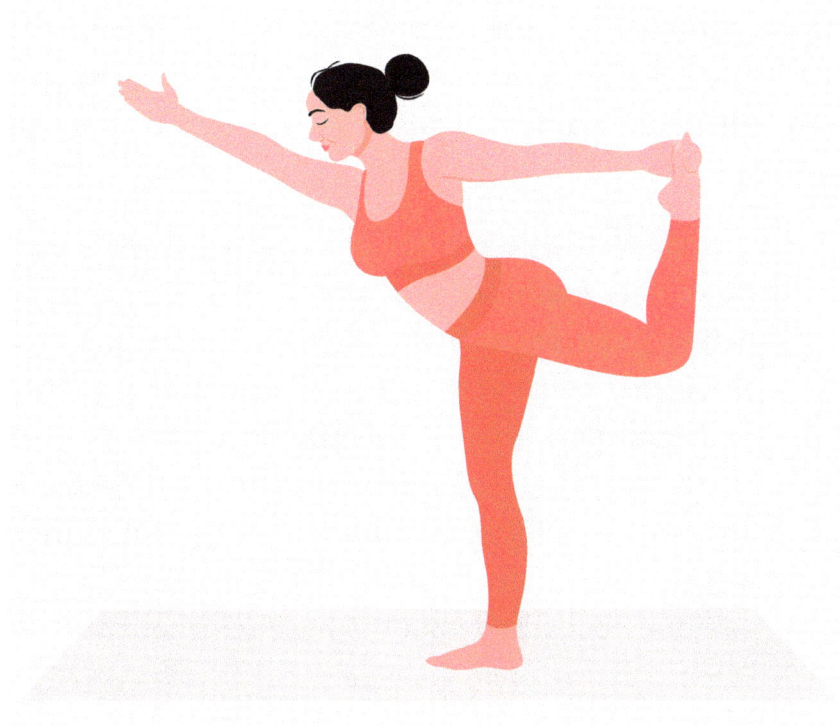

MOVE WITH MEANING

You warmed up your balance and concentration with eagle pose; now you are ready to fly. It's time for the challenging dancer's pose, where you show your might and muscle. It takes grit and focus to hold this invigorating pose, but it's something you have in spades. You are strong and confident. You know yourself. You can live large as the wonderful woman that you are. Trust your abilities. You've got this.

1. Stand up straight and pull one knee up to waist level so you are resting on one foot.
2. Suck in your stomach and find your balance.
3. Bring your bent leg back behind you. Grab your foot with the same side hand as you tip slightly forward.
4. Bend your back and stretch both arms straight, one behind you holding your foot, the other out in front of you.
5. Breathe deeply and hold the pose for a count of ten.
6. Repeat on the opposite side.

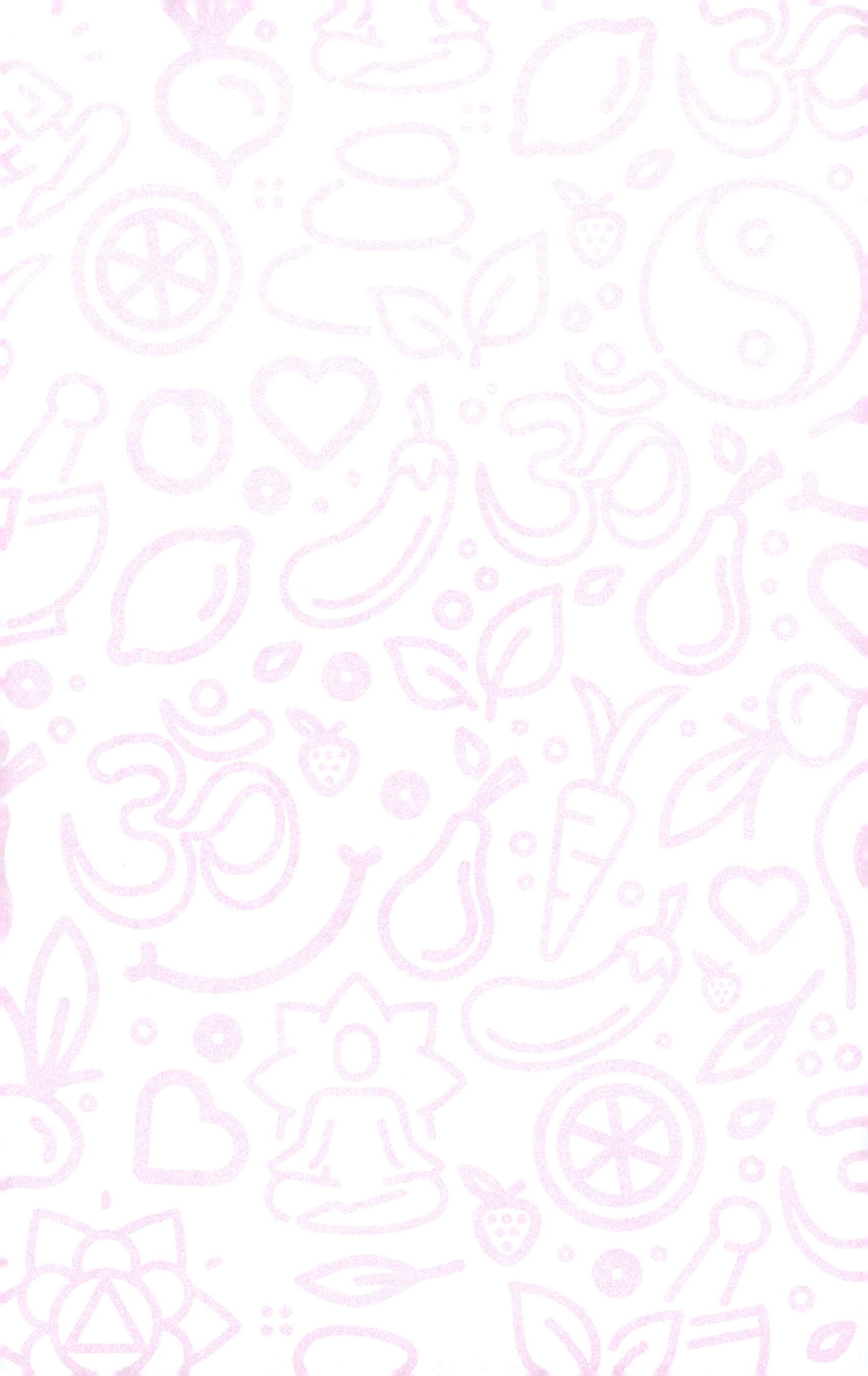

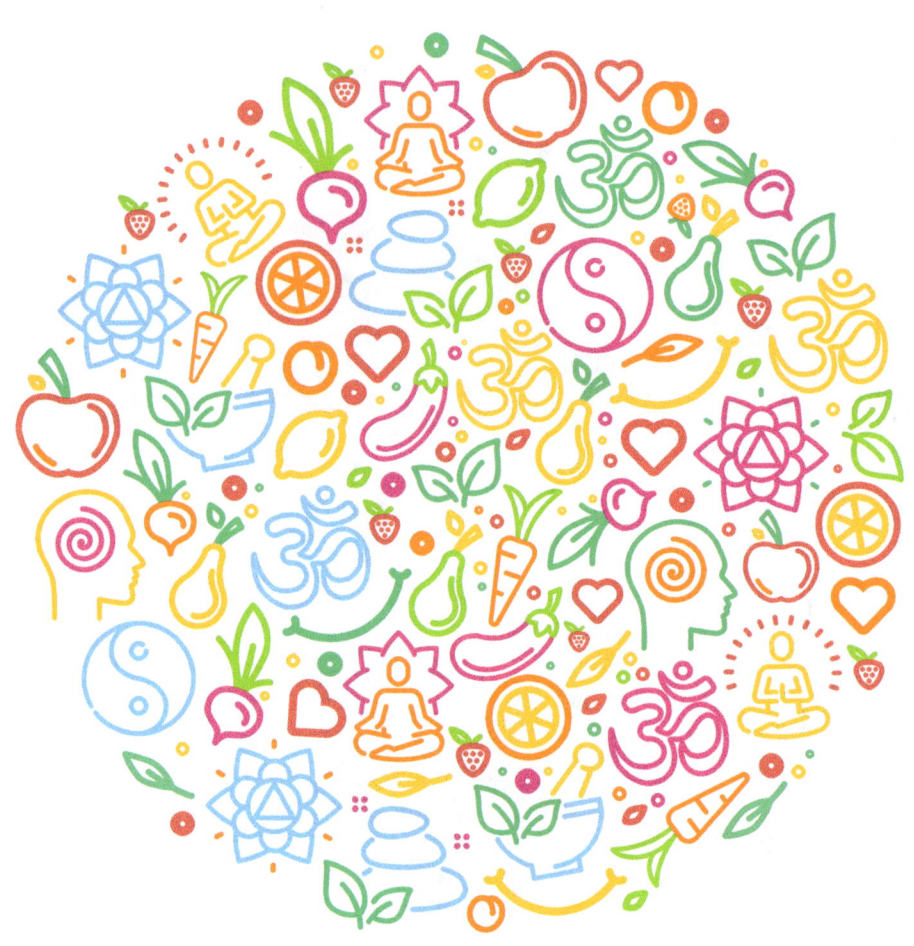

CHAPTER 7

Dining with Others

*Shimmy with Your Friends over
Shishito Peppers with White Sauce*

Remember how all-you-can-eat buffets held such appeal when you were a kid? It was like being in Willy Wonka's chocolate factory. As a family, we always celebrated Easter with the tradition of a Sunday brunch. One year, we drove to Washington, DC, for a special weekend that culminated in brunch. It was a huge spread, complete with chocolate bunnies of all sizes. I ate everything in sight. At the age of twelve, I was becoming body conscious, and I knew the connection between eating too much and gaining weight all too well. My grandfather liked to remind us to not overeat or not let ourselves go. The guilt set in once we were all in our rooms packing up our bags to go home. Everyone wondered what was taking me so long. I was in my hotel room doing leg lifts in a desperate effort to burn off some of the thousands of calories that I consumed.

That funny yet telling experience was a bit of a launch into becoming a small-scale closet eater. Some people hate to eat in front of others. They eat a tiny salad while they are out, and then when they get home, they are so hungry that they stuff themselves right before bed. I understand the psychology of closet eating. When you are ashamed of eating, you want to hide the food you eat from others. Eating in front of friends can feel uncomfortable because it's associated with shame. In other words, along the way, eating became defined as bad.

Through the years, I have consciously worked on developing a healthy relationship with food both in public and in private. For a while, I had to force myself to order what I wanted and eat. Now, if I am out with friends or family enjoying myself, I am okay with indulging a bit more than usual. I know that I can get back on track with healthy eating and healthy portions the next day.

Life is for relaxing and enjoying the moment, and that includes eating. It's not to say we should have carte blanche every time we go out to eat. When we don't feel deprived on an everyday basis, we are more likely to eat sensibly whether we are dining out with others or dining at home alone. That's why I like to let myself indulge a little in something that I'm craving. Take pizza, for example. If I cut my homemade Sausage and Arugula Pizza into strips and serve it as an appetizer, rather than offering whole pieces of the pie, we can all indulge a little without feeling like we are eating too much. You'll learn more about this philosophy of little indulgences to avoid big binges in chapter 9, titled "Indulge or You'll Bulge."

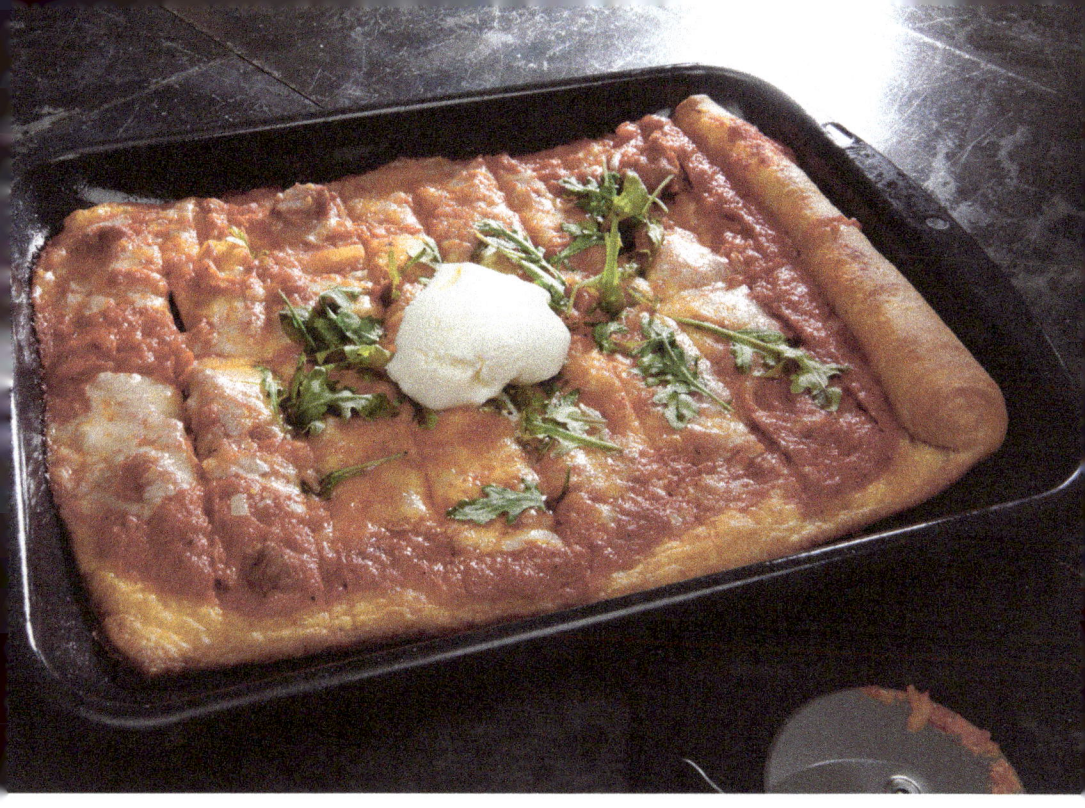

Sausage and Arugula Pizza Strips

1 crust (from store for ease)

1½ cups shredded mozzarella cheese

1 cup prepared marinara sauce (mine from chapter 5 or from a jar)

1½ cups sautéed, chopped sausage (pork or chicken, mild or spicy)

¼ cup olive oil

2 cups arugula or to taste

Brush crust with oil. Spread sauce; add cheese, then sausage. Bake at 425°F for 12 minutes. Top with arugula and serve.

We have to remember that food is fuel that our bodies rely on to function at their best. Listen to your body and be in touch with your energy level. If you are hungry, eat, no matter who you are with or no matter what time it is. Don't let the clock tell you when to eat. If you are watching your weight, eat small amounts more frequently so you don't end up starving. Moderation rules. So do my Shishito Peppers with White Sauce.

Shishito Peppers with White Sauce

1 pound shishito peppers
¼ cup olive oil
1 teaspoon sea salt

White sauce:
1 cup ranch salad dressing
1 tablespoon apple cider vinegar
½ teaspoon oregano

Place peppers in the bottom of a heated pan with oil. Add salt. Sauté until browned and softened. Mix together all white sauce ingredients and plate with peppers.

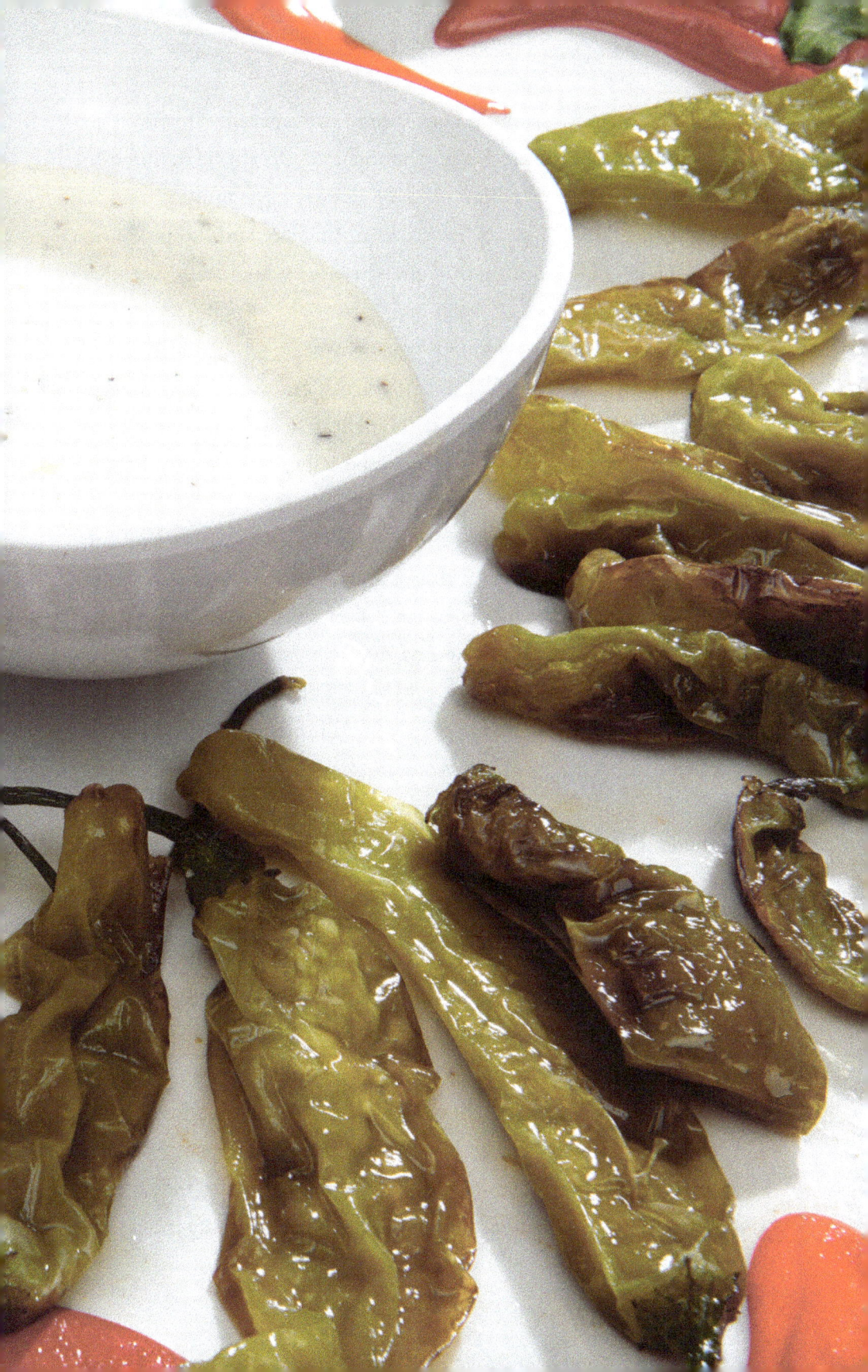

If you are trying to maintain your weight, or especially if you are in the middle of trying to lose a few pounds, you might be tempted to turn down an invite for a night out on the town with family or friends. If this is the case, I've got a few tricks up my sleeve to keep you on track. The first few require a little preplanning, which helps you stick to your plan. Here goes.

I encourage you to develop your own personal mental Rolodex (now I'm dating myself) of meals that you can order at a restaurant that are more naturally low in calories. You definitely don't have to stick to salads, but, of course, salads are one, especially simple salads that are not loaded with meat and cheese. In my Rolodex I have grilled fish, seafood, or chicken that isn't swimming in a thick white sauce (instead, opt for the red sauce, which is almost always lower in calories). Other options in my Rolodex are vegetarian dishes, sushi, and brothy soups.

Before you depart, do one of two things: Write down a few options for meal choices that fit into your diet plan on an index card or journal (or in the Notes app on your iPhone for you more tech-savvy women). Or look at the restaurant menu online beforehand and select what you will eat so that you can avoid temptation once you get there. If you get to choose the restaurant, pick one that you know has healthy items on the menu.

Another plan is "buying" calories for a favorite dish before going out. While exercise doesn't throw the door open for eating whatever you want all the time, you can use this strategy thoughtfully to give yourself leeway for special occasions. If you can make it to the gym and do the stair-climber, treadmill, or elliptical and watch those calories tick by, you can earn the chance to eat a little extra during your evening celebration, like a second cocktail or another piece of bread.

Having a plan in hand will stop the urge to order that burger and fries that the woman at the next table is enjoying way too much.

When you get home, enter what you ate in your food journal, which is just another way to hold yourself accountable. Also, focus on the conversation rather than the food. Eat slowly and engage so that you take regular pauses while eating.

As you know, I'm not one to advocate that you starve yourself. It just backfires. If you can't resist that burger, compromise by ordering it without the bun and sub a salad for the fries. There are always ways to cut out calories, like getting sauces and dressings on the side and foregoing sweet drinks for water (or a crisp wine) instead. If someone at the table is also watching her weight (and she's a good enough friend to ask), split a meal and ask the waitstaff to divide it onto two plates.

I love to plan parties and family gatherings because everything revolves around food, and if you haven't noticed by now, I love food. I literally have hundreds of recipes besides what is in this book. Making food and sharing food is my sweet spot. My mind is constantly spinning out new recipes. Like I've said, food is love and love is family.

What's great about hosting a party is that you get so busy making the food you burn calories doing it! Plus, you get to control the menu and serve healthy options, like my Pesto Shrimp appetizer. I give you a primer on party planning in chapter 11, so get excited! Notice how I include tasty ingredients, like nuts, even though they are high in calories? It's a trick of mine. Adding in a small amount of a flavorful item helps food feel indulgent. You get all the interesting flavors without the heaviness.

> If you want more of my inventive, fun, healthy, and often low-cal recipes, check out my website at officialmariasabando.com or follow me on Instagram @mariacsabando.

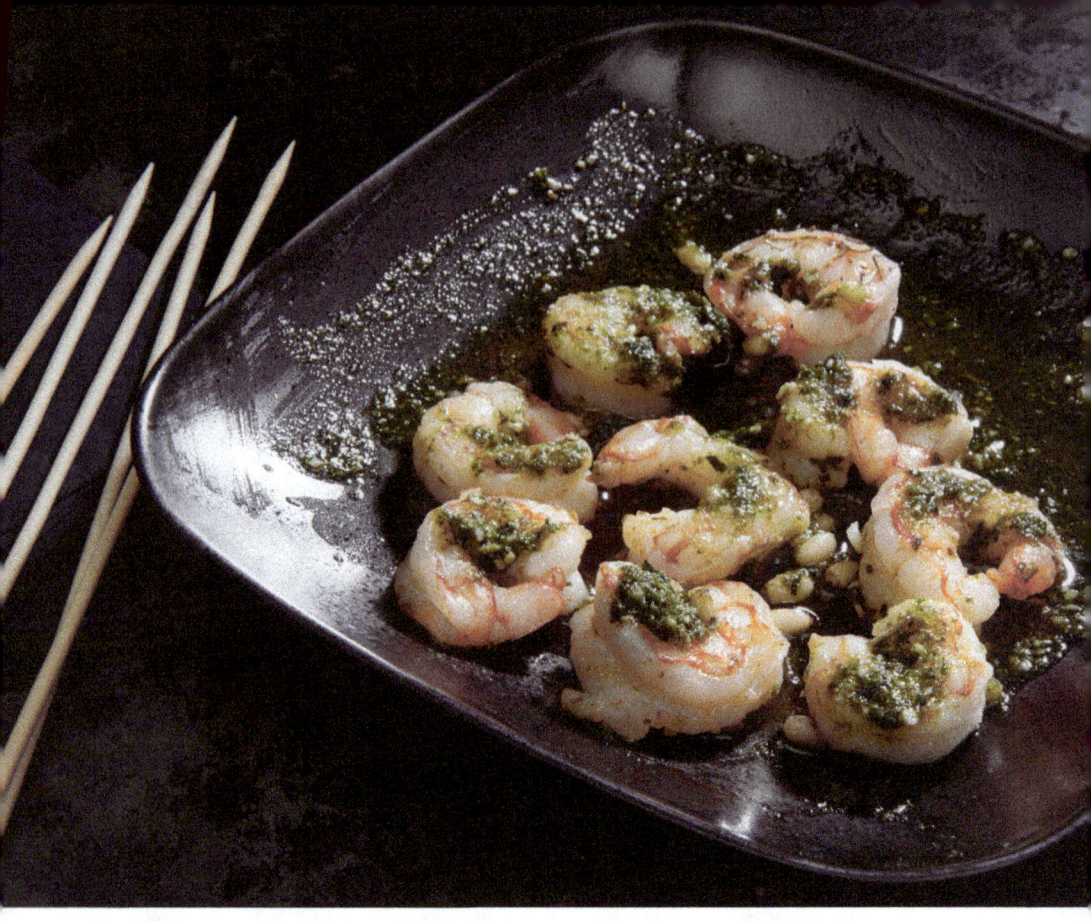

Pesto Shrimp

> 1 cup shrimp, thawed and deveined
> 1 bunch basil
> ¼ cup pistachios
> ¼ cup chopped walnuts
> 1 cup olive oil
> ½ teaspoon salt

Grill the shrimp on a grill pan with 1 teaspoon of oil. Puree the basil, walnuts, olive oil, and salt in a blender. Plate pesto and place shrimp and pistachios on top. Tip: You can make this for dinner by serving it over rice or pasta.

I totally get the urge to occasionally diet. It's a great solution for when you want to lose weight for a special event, like your daughter's wedding, but maintaining a strict diet long term and never feeling satisfied with your weight is a trap. While I don't approve of crash dieting, I do appreciate goal-oriented dieting, which you can read more about in chapter 10, where I give you a sample diet to help you lose weight over a two-week period.

Yet if your motivation to diet comes from comparing yourself to others or when you look at photos from your past when you looked your best, like at your wedding, step back and reconsider. We all get nostalgic for how we looked in the past now and then. Why do we do that to ourselves? Is it because we want to step into a time machine and go back to being that young person? Is it a desire to relive our youth, or is it a fear of growing older?

Turning back the clock is a nice first thought, but when you really think about it, you are in such a better place now. You no longer have to figure out who you are or think you should be someone different than yourself. By really examining this desire to be young again, I've learned that I really don't want to turn back the clock, not even to be the weight I was long ago.

Shake hands with food. Make food your friend, not your foe.

Happiness is about so much more than how you look in the mirror. Hopefully, when you look in the mirror before leaving for a night out on the town, you like what you see. Try not to say, "I look bad," "I wish my stomach was smaller," or "My arms are so flabby." It will only start you on a negative cycle that could lead to overeating or giving up on maintaining your health. Instead, stand in front of the mirror and force yourself to smile. While you do, make one positive comment about your looks. It sounds crazy, but it works.

Besides, feeling good about how you look does wonders for keeping the flames burning between you and your partner. In the next chapter, we'll explore ways to breathe new life into a long marriage or relationship and get back in touch with those two crazy kids who fell in love way back when.

DINING WITH OTHERS

PRAYER POSE

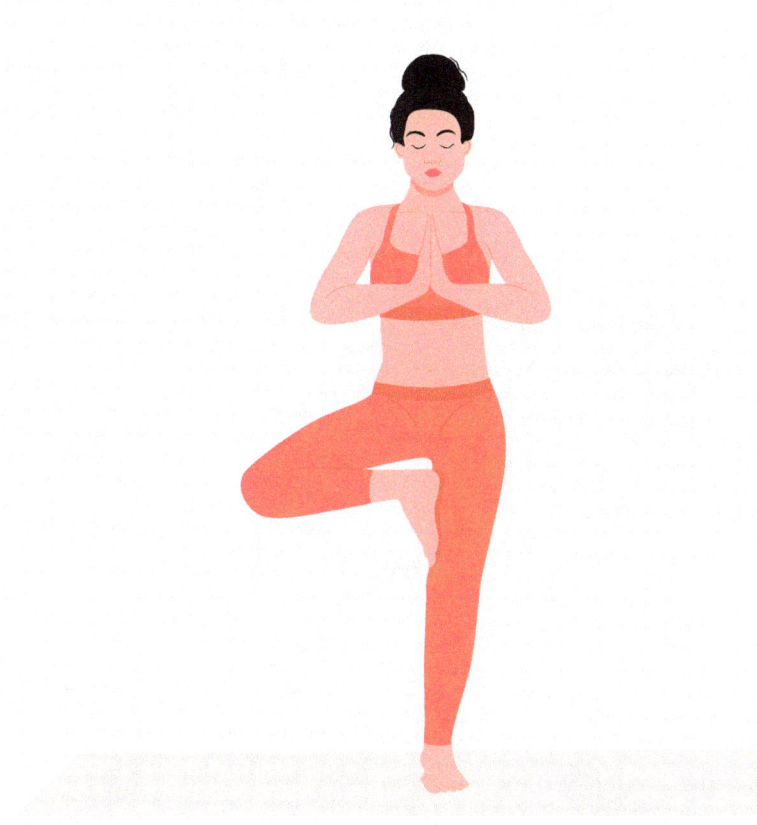

MOVE WITH MEANING

It's time to steady yourself after dancer's pose with prayer pose. Prayer pose brings you back to center while still requiring balance and effort. It's a way to pay respect to yourself and your efforts toward self-improvement. You are well on your way to living your best life in your fifties. Come into your core being and honor yourself—who you were, who you are, and who you are becoming.

1. Stand up straight and put your foot on the inner thigh of your opposite leg.
2. Press your palms together in front of your chest in a prayer position.
3. Keep your elbows even and in a straight line.
4. Stand strong and take five deep, peace-filled breaths.

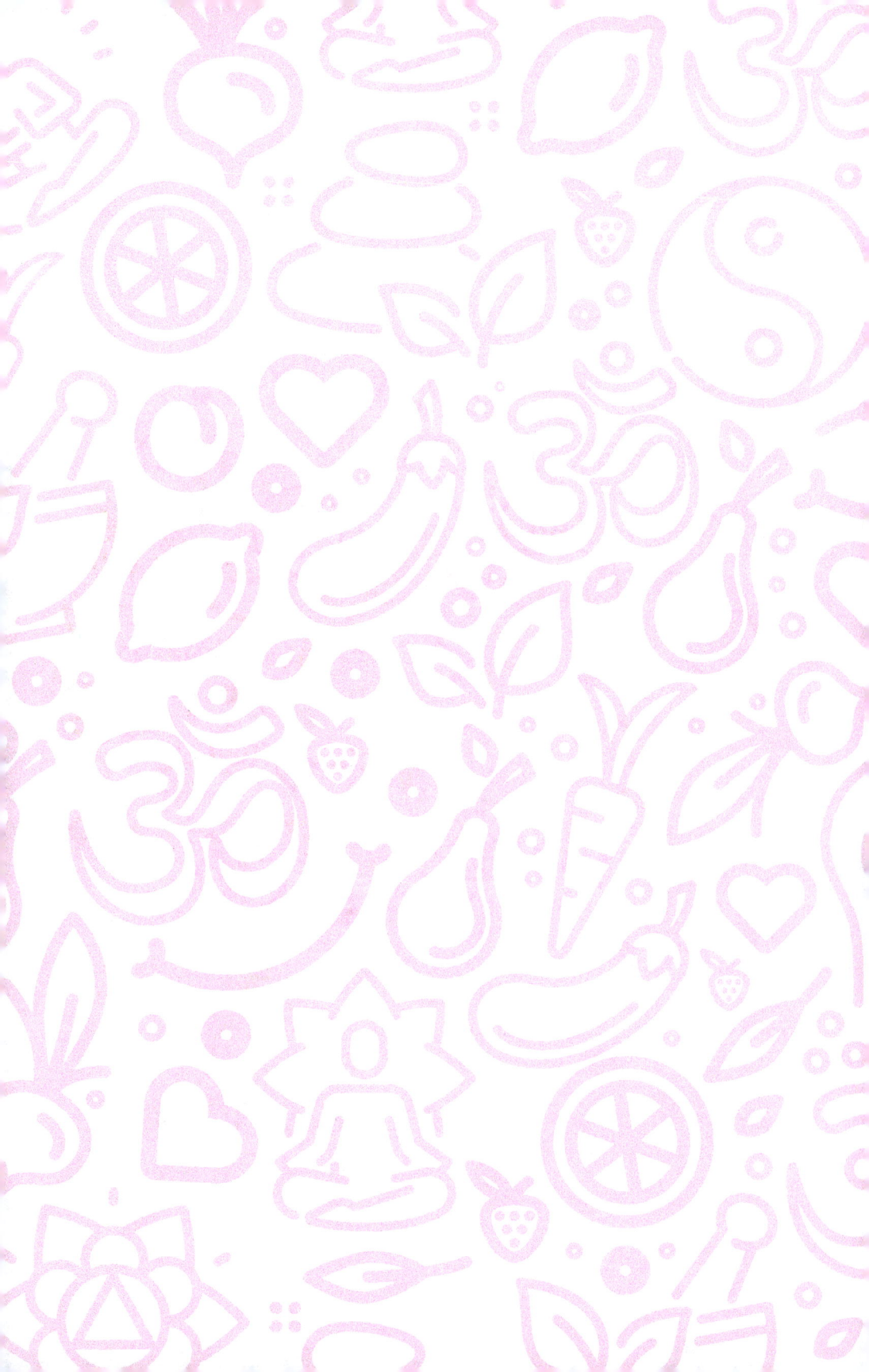

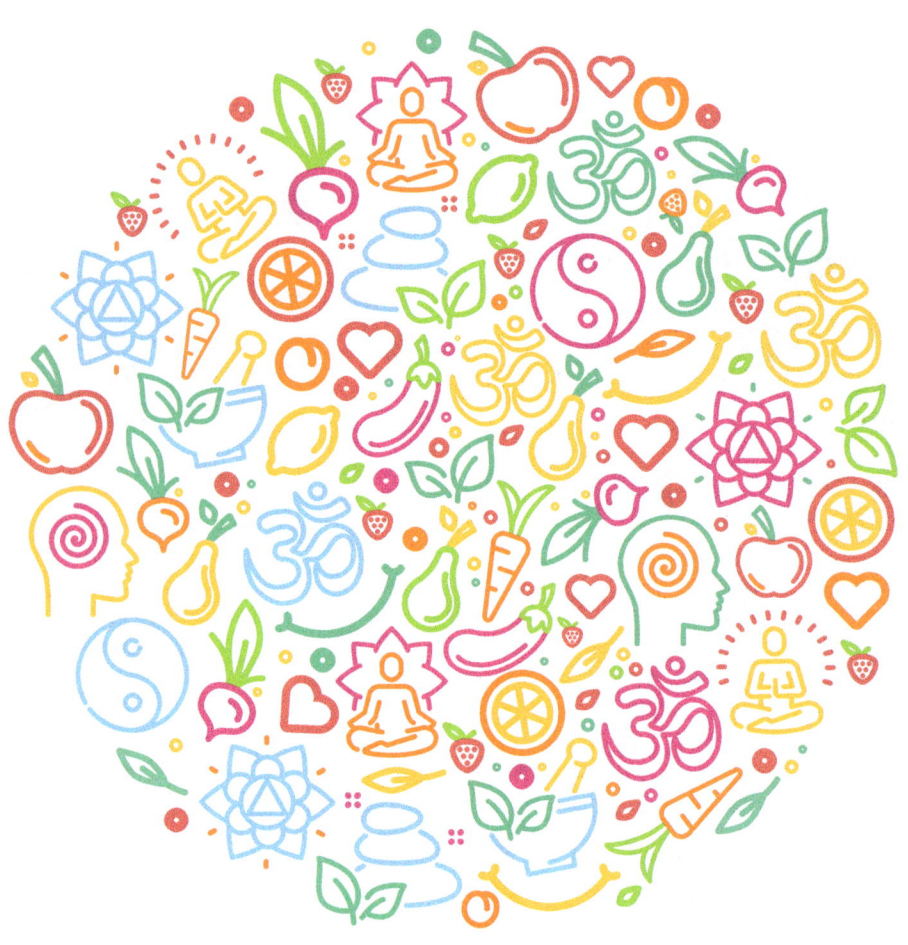

CHAPTER 8

Keep the Flames Burning
Create Some Heat with Gazpacho Shots

My Otto, he homed in on a way to keep the romance going, and he puts it on repeat like a favorite song. Along the way on our long and lovely road of marriage, he learned that I like chocolate-covered strawberries. Now, no matter what the special occasion—a romantic weekend away, a Valentine's Day celebration, or our anniversary—it's always champagne and chocolate-covered strawberries. They are sweet, but his efforts and desire to please me are even sweeter. It makes me want to heat things up with my Gazpacho Shots.

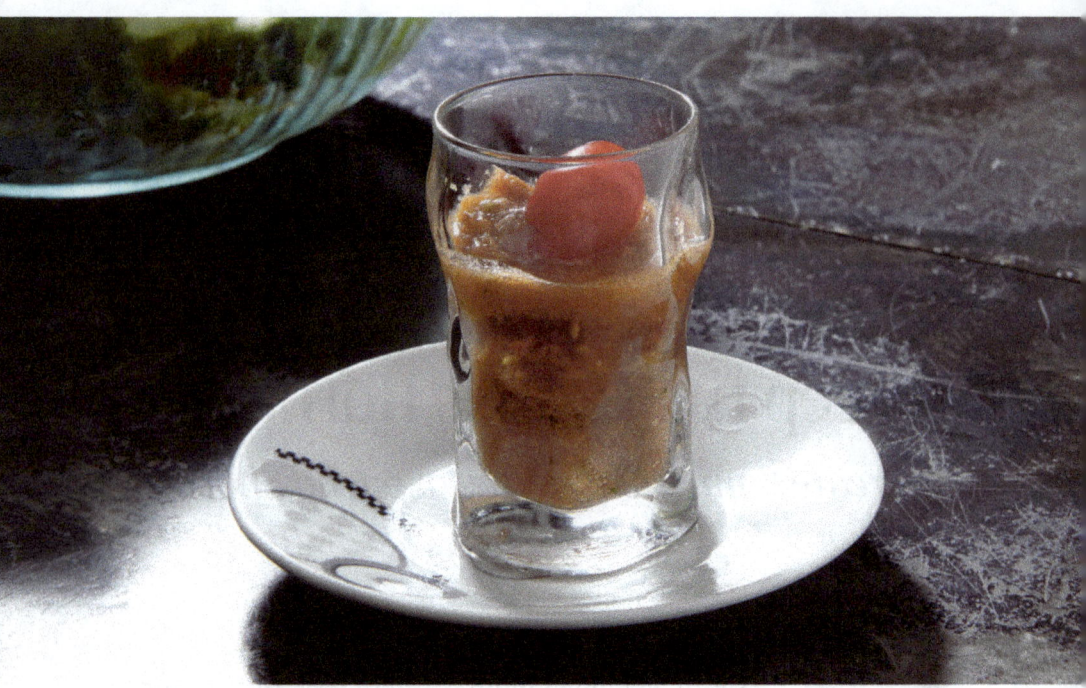

Gazpacho Shots

½ cup chopped cucumbers
½ cup cherry tomatoes
½ cup chopped bell peppers
1 teaspoon olive oil
½ teaspoon salt
Tabasco to taste, optional

Puree in blender. Pour into individual shot glasses. Toast your partner!

This chapter focuses on maintaining a healthy relationship with your husband or partner, but if you don't have one right now, don't skip ahead! Many of the same guidelines I suggest here apply to every relationship in your life. There are a lot of ways to keep the flames of your relationships burning, and some of it starts in the kitchen. We've all heard the old saying "The way to a husband's heart is through his stomach." I say it applies to more than your husband, but mine certainly appreciates the love I put into a home-cooked meal. It's an idea I absorbed from the Italian women in my family and an idea that's reinforced in the grateful faces smiling back at me from around the table, then and now. Cooking is an act of love and a great way to express your caring for your spouse.

The next time you are looking for a new recipe (like on my website at officialmariasabando.com), first consider what ingredients your husband enjoys. Even if, say, jalapeños are not your favorite food, find a recipe that sounds delicious that you can make to please him. I'm not advocating that you return to the 1950s and please your man at all costs and all the time. I am advocating that you cook with your partner in mind, which will infuse the meal—and the sentiment—with love. Making sure to put your partner's needs first at times is vital for a healthy relationship.

Relationships are more a labor of love than hard labor.

Here is more relationship advice that might surprise you: the secret ingredient to a healthy marriage is humor. And I'm not talking about just a little humor now and then. I mean your whole relationship should be centered around humor. Of course, the assumption is that you have attraction and fondness or you wouldn't have ended up together, but maintaining a long-term relationship demands enjoyment, and nothing gets you there faster than humor. Think about it. Your closest relationships have inside jokes and innuendos, and intimacy is often born out of teasing, shared secrets, and sweet yet silly nicknames. They make you feel like you are in a secret club. They help you let loose and feel human and alive.

If you lose humor in a relationship, you lose everything. My husband has a good sense of humor; it's nice and dry like a glass of sauvignon blanc. My humor is a little more edgy and ironic, but no matter who is slinging the jokes, it's bonding. Plus, life is too serious as it is. Couples have to worry about finances, fixing cars, caring for kids (or grandkids), maintaining the house, etc., etc., etc. Like I say, if you are not laughing, you are crying. Also, keeping things playful is downright sexy. Do you know what else is playful and sexy? My White Sangria Spritzer. Just be careful: a little wine helps you feel romantic, but since we are older, your chance for a hangover is greater; it's irony at play when you want to get romantic, isn't it?!

White Sangria Spritzer

5 grapes (or a handful of blueberries or orange slices)
7 ounces white wine, any type
1 ounce seltzer or ginger ale

Combine seltzer/soda and wine. Add ice, if desired. Drop in the grapes. Makes 1 serving. Double as needed.

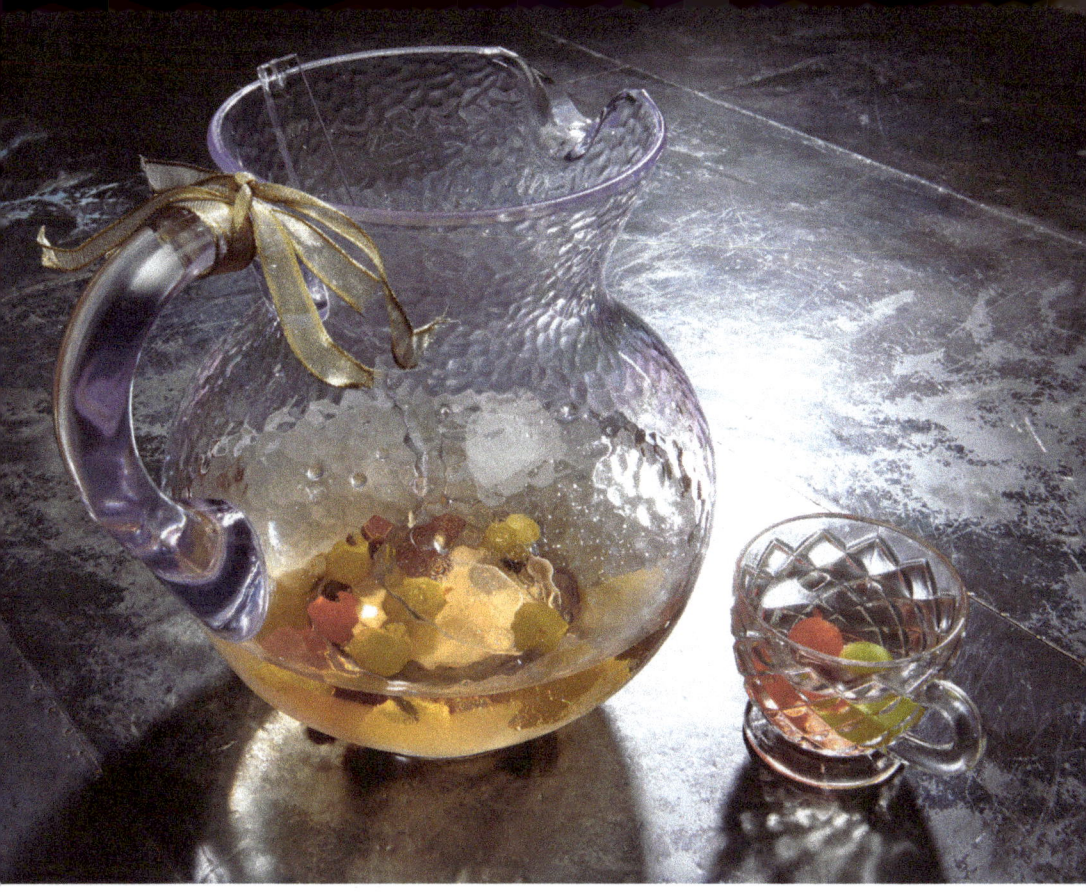

The second most important ingredient in a healthy marriage is communication. This goes for everyone in your life—your sister, brother, parents, spouse, kids, friends, and coworkers. Remember when I talked about how we have to stay vulnerable to become the best versions of ourselves? When we are dishonest with our partner and unwilling to talk about our concerns or problems, we shut out the chance to get close. Same goes for when we carry resentments until we've built a wall, brick by unyielding brick. Ask yourself, "What makes me happier? To have a nice, solid wall or a close relationship?"

I get it. It's harder to communicate honestly than it is to fabricate and hide. At least in the short run. But it is better to take the fallout or feel the heat than to deny the real you. If you are continually sweeping dirt under the rug, it's going to get lumpy, and you are going to trip and fall. But you're in your fifties, and I know you are wise and you know all this. You probably give your friends the same advice! Seeing things clearly is hard from the inside of your own relationship, but if there are unresolved issues in your marriage, it's never too late to clear the air. And if you need help doing that, by all means ask for help.

Good communication is easier said than done, but hey, what in life isn't? Remember to compromise and meet your partner halfway. Set down your defenses and listen. You can repair hurtful things by being your loving, open self. I truly believe that the more you give, the more you get back. What's great about open communication is that it helps build intimacy. The closer you feel to your partner, the more self-accepting you become of your own body because you trust that your significant other loves you just the way you are. That all adds up to you loving your own body more and accepting it even if it has changed over the years (of course it has, and that's okay!). I love the idea of couples aging well together and growing old with complete comfort and understanding.

ACTIVE LISTENING FOR BETTER COMMUNICATION

We think of listening as passive, but good listening is active. It takes concentration, patience, and respect. It's a therapy method of giving someone your full attention and then reflecting back to them what they are saying. You are not thinking about what you will say when it's your turn to speak. You are not judging what they say. Instead, you are in the moment with your partner, trying to understand his perspective. Consider making a regular date for this turn-taking exercise. Maybe it's a nightly check-in before you turn off the lights. Maybe it's a Saturday morning ritual over coffee. If you are sharing something hard or addressing a concern, do so from the "I" point of view rather than pointing the finger with a "you." Ask for clarification on whether or not your perception is correct, and allow your partner to answer without any preconceived ideas. It's easy to think we know our long-term spouse completely, but people grow and change, and we need to be open to each other's new ways of being.

Sometimes we need therapy to get over a hump. Therapy works because it's like having someone at your side, encouraging you without judgment to be your best married self. It makes you aware of not only your own needs but also your partner's needs. It creates a third person at the table—your relationship. You both meet halfway to feed the relationship. People think therapy has a bad connotation, that it makes you look weak. That's old-school thinking. In reality, it makes you look strong. And remember, it can be short term if you just need a tune-up or to hit the reset button.

Do you know the Black Eyed Peas song "Meet Me Halfway"?[15] Its chorus runs through my head when I think about my marriage. It's a good reminder to honor each other's needs and keep the relationship equal. A one-sided relationship never works! The song goes: "Can you meet me halfway (I'll meet you halfway)? Right at the borderline, that's where I'm gonna wait for you. I'll be looking out, night 'n' day. Took my heart to the limit, and this is where I'll stay." Another thing

---

15 "The Black Eyed Peas—Meet Me Halfway (Official Music Video)," accessed June 15, 2022, https://www.youtube.com/watch?v=I7HahVwYpwo.

that takes people's hearts to the limit is my Maria's Bloody Mary. Try one during a spontaneous weekend couple's brunch!

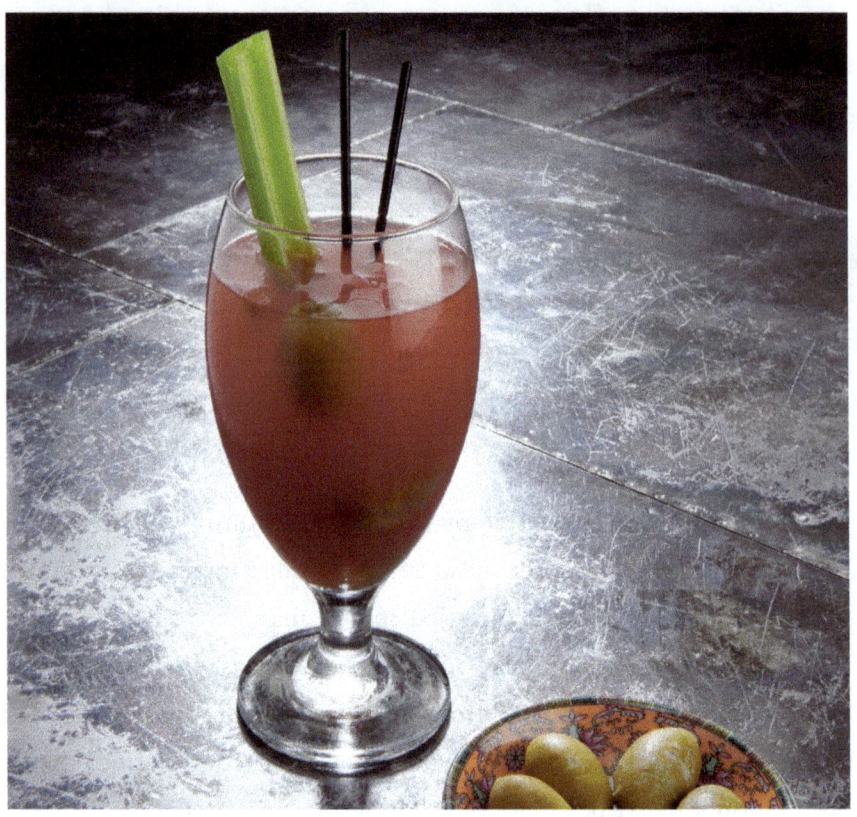

Maria's Bloody Mary

- 8 ounces tomato juice
- 1 ounce vodka
- 3 large Spanish olives
- 1 stalk celery
- 1 teaspoon Worcestershire sauce

Combine juice, vodka, and Worcestershire sauce. Garnish with olives and celery stalk. Cheers!

Regarding communication, here's one more word of advice. Don't assume your spouse knows everything about you, even if you have been together for decades. The word "negotiation" is an unattractive word for romance, but the ability to peacefully negotiate, and compromise, keeps couples moving along comfortably. The same is true for compassion and having the willingness to take the wheel when your partner can't.

In church, I recently heard the priest talk about marriage as a boat. Sometimes it's your partner who is drowning and needs rescuing, or he needs to take a break from paddling or steering and simply float. You have to jump in and take over, because there will be times in the future when you need rescuing or a break. You act because you love your partner and you want to be there to catch them, and you know they will do the same for you.

With long marriages, it can be easy to take each other for granted. We assume that our spouse will stick by us no matter what. Yet without nourishment, relationships wither. Be kind. Be supportive. Be respectful. Marriage is a labor of love. Treat your spouse like you do your best friend, with the same polite listening, gentle guidance, acceptance, and forgiveness.

Enough seriousness—it's time to lighten up! Let's talk about planning a date night, a nice easy-breezy celebration of your union. The plan is to have no strict plan, just a fun, loose get-together so that there is no pressure, letting spontaneity rule the evening! If you have expectations, they might fall flat, and the last thing you want is disappointment.

If your date night is a quiet, romantic night at home, keep the menu super simple so you are rested and relaxed for your date. Try my simple and light Twisted Lemon Cocktail with a few decadent appetizers. Set a nice table with lots of candles, low lighting, and a favorite musician that you both love playing on the stereo.

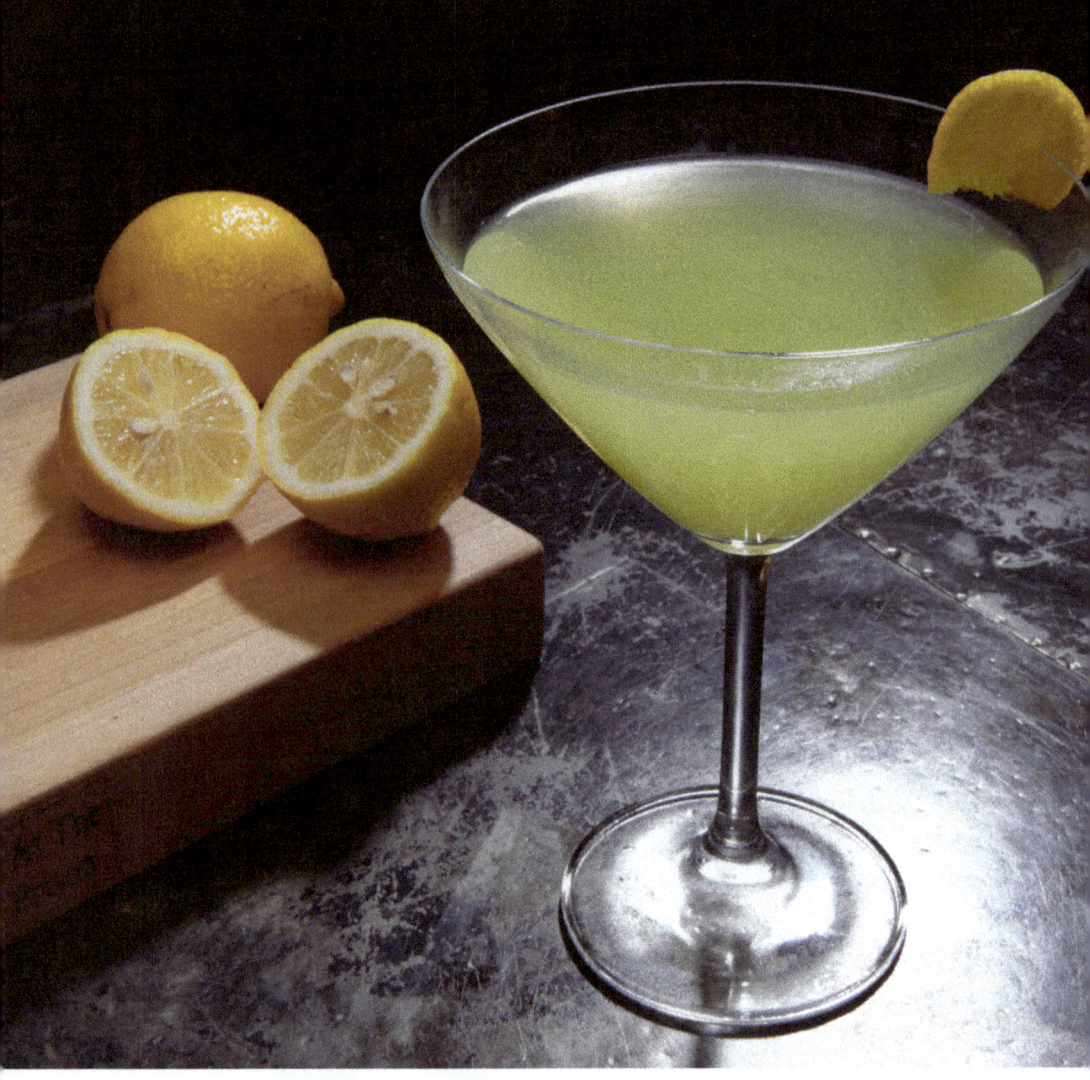

Twisted Lemon Cocktail

- 1 ounce vodka
- 1 cup prepared lemonade
- 1 lemon rind for garnish
- Ice (optional)

Pour vodka and lemonade over ice and stir. Garnish with lemon rind.

Sometimes it's easier to connect when you are away from home, where reminders of all the house projects and daily tasks are gone. Ironically, it is sometimes your marriage that takes the back seat to all your other responsibilities, and that can impact your relationship both emotionally and physically. A wonderful way to bond is to dream together. Is there something you both want to do that can go on your mutual bucket list? Like someday visiting a foreign country together? There's great unity in achieving dreams together. My husband and I have had a dream of taking our girls to Italy and bonding over delicious sights, sounds, and, of course, food. I am happy to say that we finally made that dream come true, and it was better than I ever could have dreamed.

If you can't plan a big trip right now, plan a fun date. Get creative and use your imagination! How about dinner and minigolf, or a day at an amusement park? For a fun twist, try a one-night getaway in your own town where you play tourist and try new restaurants and venues, ending with a night at a hotel. Or splurge on a beach vacation, just you two. Having adventures together is bonding. So is finding activities that you both enjoy doing and doing them regularly, together. It all helps you tap into your core connection and attraction that you had when you first met. Those young kids are still in you! Encourage them to come out and have some fun.

Besides communication, compassion, and compromise, marriage is about connection—the physical kind! In fact, I'd say the first three Cs add up to about 50 percent of what makes a happy marriage. Physical connection is the other half. I'm no Dr. Ruth, but it's what I believe, and I stand by it. Physical touch is the driver for the other three. When you make it a part of your daily ritual within your relationship to give a hug for no reason, a grab of the hand, or an unexpected goodbye kiss, it is a warm little exchange that reminds you both that you love each other. Think of these little physical connections as chocolate kisses that melt in your mouth and make you feel delicious.

You've gotten the message loud and clear by now that keeping the flames burning requires spontaneity, flexibility, and staying open to new ideas and activities. It's the same with maintaining a healthy lifestyle. Too many rules and rigidity with relationships, food, or exercise often backfires. In the next chapter, I introduce you to one of my favorite mantras—indulge or you'll bulge. It softens the corners of your weight-management plan, letting you know that it's okay to indulge sometimes, and you can do it completely guilt-free.

SIDE PLANK

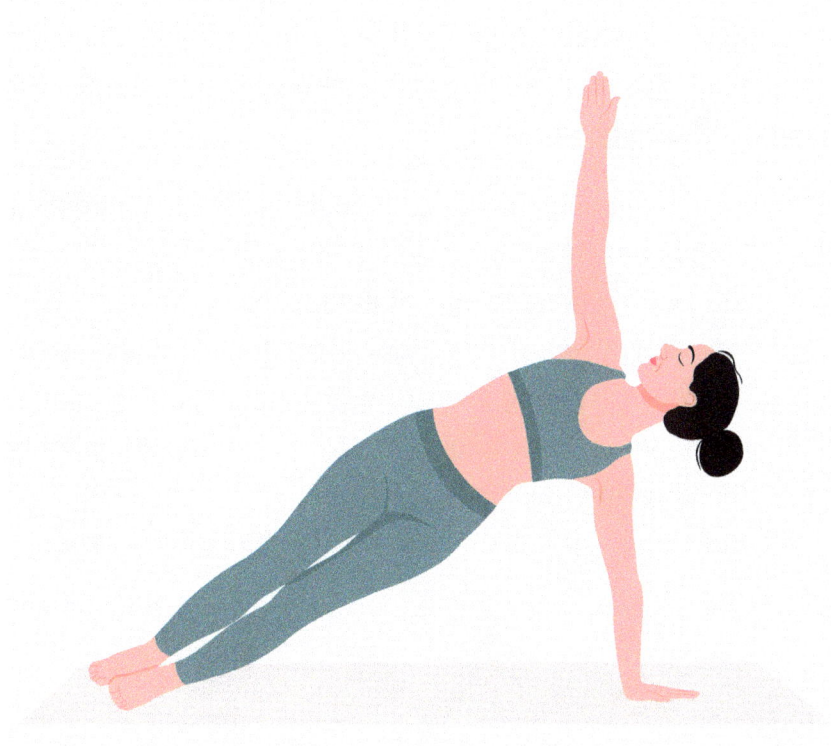

MOVE WITH MEANING

Having connected with your partner, you move from the stable prayer pose down to the floor for a side plank. It's time to feel the burn! Planks are difficult moves that demand concentration. You put a lot in, and you get a lot out, just like with a healthy relationship. It's work, but it's also oh so satisfying.

1. Lie on your side, leaning on the forearm that's resting steadily on the floor.
2. Stack your legs on top of each other.
3. Lift your hips off the ground so that all your weight is on your resting bent arm and your resting foot.
4. Raise your opposite arm up above your head or place it on your hip.
5. Hold the plank for thirty to forty-five seconds.

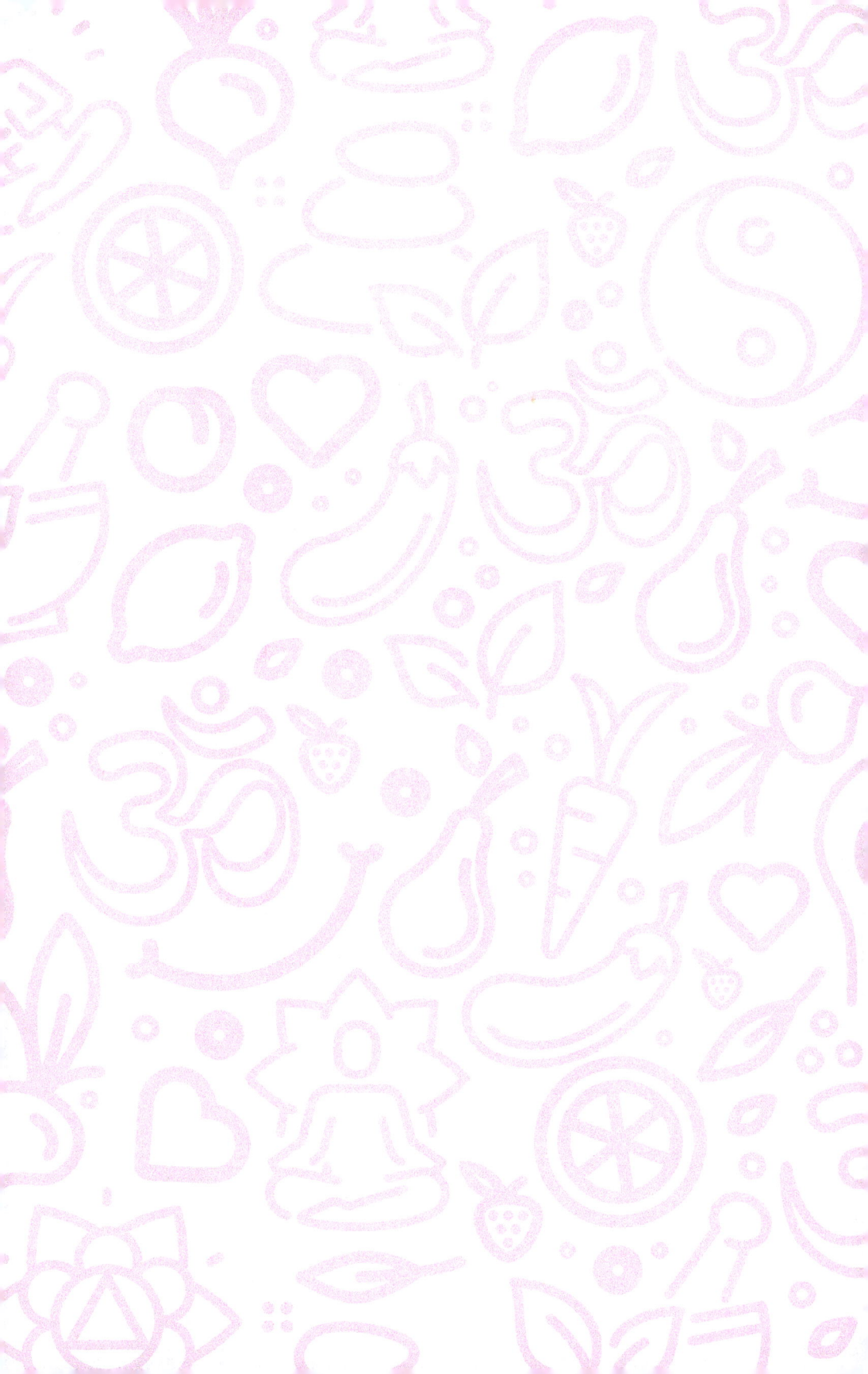

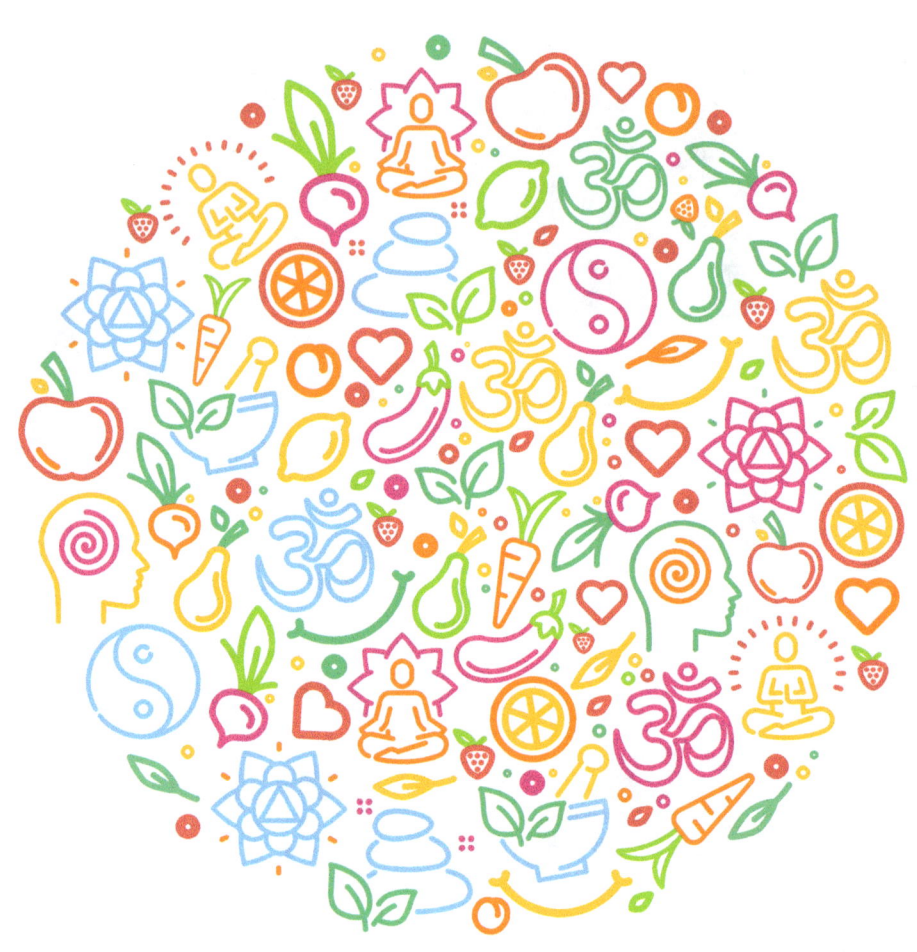

CHAPTER 9

Indulge or You'll Bulge

*Mollify Your Munchies with a
Little Mac 'n' Cheese Supreme*

When I was in my early teens, I was always trying new diets. I loved reading, so I would go to the library in the summer and check out a ton of books. I remember sitting outside with my sister with a pile of books spread out all around me—books on dieting, on exercise, and on cooking (kind of funny how those exact interests are what my book is about today). I was at that tender age when you become aware of your body, and like most observant girls who came of age in the '80s, I got the message from society that thin was in.

One of the cookbooks that I read talked about cooking without a drop of oil or salt. I thought it was brilliant. I went straight into the kitchen, where my mom was cooking dinner, to share what I learned, thinking she would be astounded. To my surprise, she wasn't impressed. She merely said, "It's really hard to make good food without oil or salt." And she's right, of course. Little did I know that cooking involves a balance between enjoying yummy food and staying healthy. So our focus should be low fat, not nonfat. Mom was always right; I just didn't see it until I was much older!

I dabbled in dieting throughout high school, and when I went to college and heard about the freshman fifteen (the fifteen pounds freshman girls were predicted to gain), I vowed that would not be me. I doubled down on dieting and lost weight instead of gaining it. Maybe you can relate. Thankfully, I was able to see that this strategy wasn't healthy. I kind of did that yo-yo thing and gained the weight I'd lost back, plus the freshman fifteen! Looking back, I laugh at the irony of that.

During that phase as a college freshman, I had become disconnected from reality when it came to food. Just the other day, my sister and I were talking about all the funny things that happened in our past. She said, "Maria, I remember when you said anyone who ate lunch was an extremely weak person." Can you imagine? Let my story help you stop pining for your youth and rather help you find gratitude for being the wise fiftysomething woman that you are today! I loved my youth, but I don't want to go back there and relive it. As we age, our idea of food shifts; hopefully from an archenemy to a kind friend who is offering nourishment for our bodies.

> **Allowing yourself to indulge a little along the way satisfies your cravings and helps you stay on track with your weight-management goals.**

The big lesson from my crazy youth is that when we make food—or anything, for that matter—too black and white, we set ourselves up for failure. There are not two bins in front of us—a black one for "bad" food and a white one for "good" food. There is just food, and there is just us. Life exists in the gray. I admit sometimes this is hard for me. Gray is messy and complicated, but it's real. Saying I am going to be "good" all of the time with what I eat and never saying, "Forget it—I will eat and drink whatever I want!" used to set me up for a binge session. I've learned through the years that if I drop the all-or-nothing mentality, I have more success. Living in the gray is more real because we are human. We don't always do what's best for us, our moods do affect what we eat, and being flexible with ourselves helps us give an inch instead of taking a mile.

So, now and then, or on special occasions, allow yourself a taste of honey, whether your honey is a cupcake or a small serving of my easy but oh-so-yummy Mac 'n' Cheese Supreme!

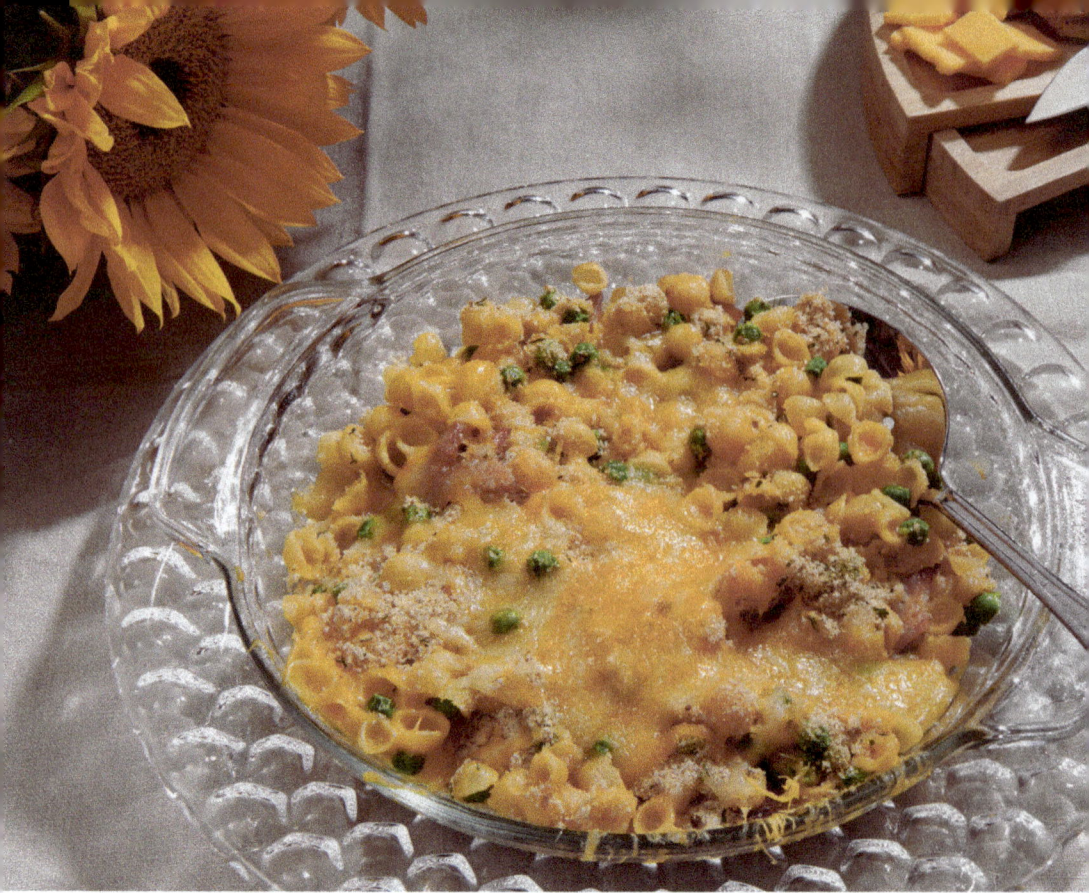

Mac 'n' Cheese Supreme

> 2 boxes prepared macaroni and cheese
> ¼ cup cream or whole milk
> ½ cup bread crumbs
> 2 strips bacon, fried until crispy, finely chopped
> ½ cup shredded cheddar cheese
> 1 bag frozen peas

Prepare macaroni and cheese according to package instructions (use butter option). Combine with all additional ingredients except for bread crumbs. Top with bread crumbs and bake at 350°F for 15 minutes. Also a great side dish!

My philosophy today is that if you don't let yourself cheat once in a while, you are going to feel deprived, and you'll go off the deep end. It's better to blow your weight-management plan just a little bit—one day or one meal at a time. As long as it's the exception and you can get back on track without completely giving up, you are good to go. So the next time you are really craving a scoop of ice cream at a birthday party, and it's not a usual treat, go for it. Just live in the gray while you do it. What I mean by that is ask for a kiddie scoop or a single scoop and skip all the toppings. Then, sit down guilt-free and savor every bite.

Some women swear by a cheat day. They stick to a diet or weight-management plan for a week or two, then one day they let themselves eat whatever they want. If you think it would work for you, go for it! I'm not a huge fan of cheat days. I would rather eat moderately over the week with an occasional treat rather than blow it all in one day. Allowing myself a small slice of pie or a second glass of wine while staying on track otherwise on a day-to-day basis is more my style. But you know your style. You've come this far, and you know what works for you and what doesn't. Listen to that wise voice inside of you—the one that sounds calm and reasonable—and commit to doing what it says. You know you, so just do *you*!

You don't have to be thin to be moody, and you don't have to be chubby to be jolly.

Indulge or you'll bulge doesn't mean eat all you want all day long. It also doesn't mean that you should stick to a strict diet only to burn out a few weeks later and start the see-food diet and eat everything in sight. It requires thoughtful pauses and ongoing conscious consideration. It's a concept that demands discernment rather than a free-for-all attitude. After all, you wake up every morning with one waistline—yours. Be choosy about indulging. For me, a piece or two of chocolate or a handful of salty potato chips is all I need to satisfy a craving. That splurge only amounts to about 100 well-spent calories. It satisfies my craving without blowing up my weight-management plan of eating just 1,500 calories a day. Living healthily in the gray zone is one of my personal mantras regarding food. What are yours?

Another goal with eating is to find that happy medium of staying satiated without feeling stuffed. Like I talked about earlier in the book, eating slowly, being conscious of enjoying your food, and listening to your body goes a long way. It comes down to lifestyle changes. When you start adopting healthy habits and sticking to them for the most part, your weight steadies out. Also, it's imperative that you decide what healthy habits work for you. This book tells you what works for me. When you read an idea, watch your reaction. If you feel it click into place, adopt it. After all, you know what works best in the long run for you. That's just it. Eating healthy is the long game and strict diets are the short game.

SAY NO TO THE YO-YO

If a diet promises that you will drastically lose weight fast, pass it right on by. That's because yo-yo dieting, going on a strict diet only to go off it later, isn't healthy. When you lose weight fast, you tend to lose muscle with the fat. You may think you did great losing five pounds in a week or two, but if you ditch the diet and go back to overeating without heavy exercise, guess what? You gain back fat, not muscle. Even if you don't care about looking muscular, it's not healthy to carry extra fat. The more muscle you have, the higher your metabolism and the more fat you burn. Another reason to say no to the yo-yo is that it is hard on your heart—and your self-esteem. Plus, certain fad diets, like eating bars or shakes, don't help you learn about healthy eating. Gaining weight back makes you feel like you failed. Instead, be a turtle and find a slow and steady diet that helps you create healthy habits with food and exercise, and you'll win the weight-management race.[16]

The battle of the bulge…for me, it has a psychological meaning, not a historical one. Although battling our weight is not life or death, it can wreak havoc with our emotions. The battle of the bulge is real, and balance is essential. Let's be sure to not beat ourselves up, because eating is a good thing, not a bad thing. So next time you hear this historical reference, try to keep it in perspective without relating it to your personal emotions around your body. Notice what you are doing right and build on that.

Let's be real. Sometimes we let loose. We eat or drink too much. If that happens, be gentle with yourself. After all, you are only human! A magnificent, beautiful human, but human. Forgive yourself and recommit. Go back to eating normally tomorrow. What throws us off is swinging to the extremes. We starve ourselves as a punishment for overindulging, or we give up completely and start a cyclone of overeating. I don't know about you, but if I starve myself, my body

---

16   Livestrong, "What Really Happens to Your Body When You Yo-Yo Diet," accessed July 6, 2022, https://www.livestrong.com/article/13720977-yo-yo-dieting-affects/.

fights back with a primitive hunger, and I set myself up for overeating. Instead, simply return to your healthy routines around eating and move on. However, if you feel indulgent, and you have a special occasion coming up, make an Italian classic, Eggplant Parmesan. Raise a glass of red vino with your family or friends and enjoy.

Eggplant Parmesan

1 eggplant, quartered

¼ cup olive oil

3 cups of my easy Italian primer sauce (page 154) or jarred pasta sauce

3 cups shredded mozzarella cheese

3 cups ricotta cheese

2 teaspoons Parmesan cheese

Boil eggplant until soft, about 20 minutes, then fry in oil. Slice the eggplant lengthwise and arrange on the bottom of a casserole dish. Top with tomato sauce. Dollop ricotta cheese on top. Top with shredded mozzarella and Parmesan cheese. Bake at 375°F for 20 minutes.

Speaking of pasta, it's about time that I share my Italian primer. Italian food is indulgent food, but that doesn't mean it has to be difficult to make. If you don't have time to make a homemade sauce, jarred spaghetti sauces work; just pick one that's low in sugar. If you want to sweeten your sauce, do it with red wine.

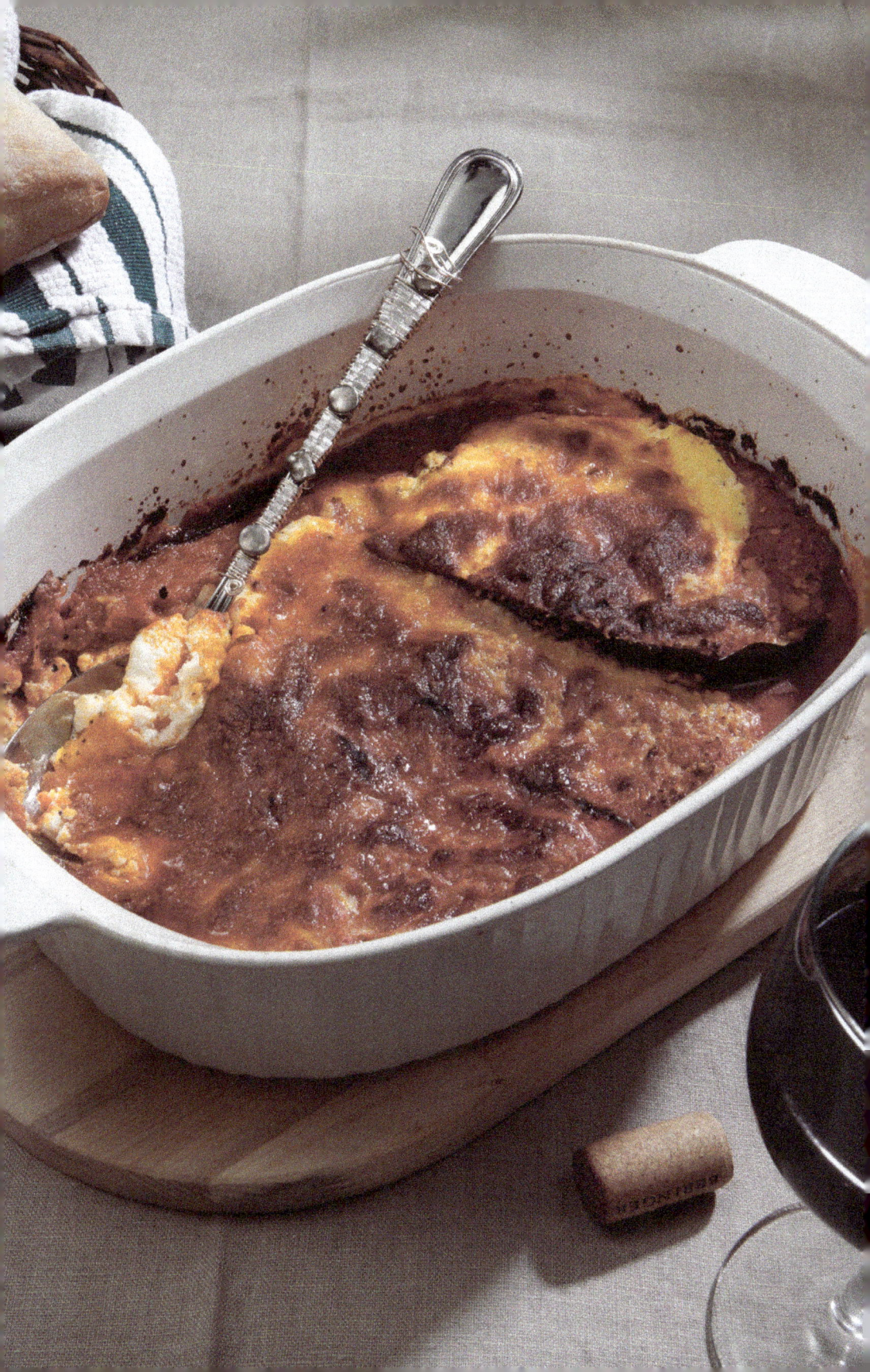

MARIA'S ITALIAN COOKING PRIMER

Follow these easy steps to make a basic Italian pasta sauce, which you can dress up as you see fit or serve as is.

1. Every one of my pan-based Italian recipes starts with a splash of olive oil in a pan.
2. When the oil is hot (but not smokin' hot!), add a few super thinly sliced garlic cloves, letting them cook for a quick half minute until they dissolve in the pan.
3. Add in meat or veggies and brown over medium heat, including chopped onions. (Skip this step if you are making simple marinara.)
4. Next come the tomatoes. Fresh is best. Cut up and mix in about one and a half pounds of fresh tomatoes or add a twenty-eight-ounce can of crushed tomatoes. You can add a few tablespoons of tomato paste to thicken your sauce if you desire.
5. Add about half a teaspoon of dried oregano (or one and a half teaspoons of fresh).
6. Simmer for about thirty minutes. Stir often with a wooden spoon.
7. While your sauce is simmering, cook your noodles. Add salt to the water to make it boil faster. I tend to go with spaghetti for marinara and ziti for meat sauce, but use whatever pasta you like. On the days that you are not indulging, try zoodles (zucchini noodles) or whole-grain pasta for a healthy alternative.

The concept of *indulge or you'll bulge* doesn't just apply to food. Indulging also applies to exercise. If you slept poorly the night before, or your workday went too long, trade in your trip to the gym for a walk outside in the fresh air instead. Or swap your exercise class for a few floor exercises or dumbbell curls at home. Better yet, if you have energy, go do an activity that you truly enjoy. Maybe it is tootling on your bike down a nearby bike path. When exercise feels indulgent, you've found the sweetest win-win around. I do yoga almost every day, some days just a few stretches and poses, other days a long, challenging workout. Yoga is both a physical and spiritual practice for me. Because I enjoy it, I do it. When I do it regularly, I'm a happier person. Find your yoga and do it every chance that you get.

Here's another mind twister. Indulging doesn't just apply to food and exercise; it applies to your *whole life*. When you let yourself indulge a little when dreaming about your future plans and envisioning the life that you want, you are more likely to live it. What feels indulgent to you? What fills you up? What do you want more of in your life? Maybe it's a day or weekend with girlfriends, drinking wine, and connecting through inside jokes and laughter. Maybe it's getting out in nature and trying your hand at capturing the perfect photograph. Maybe it's learning a new activity, like taking a martial arts class. Or how about achieving a personal challenge for yourself, like trying an open mic at the local comedy club, writing a piece of music, or picking up an instrument you played as a kid? When you work up an appetite while adventuring, and you are too busy having fun to cook, try my easy Air Fryer Chicken Tenders and Fries.

Air Fryer Chicken Tenders and Fries

Chicken tenders:
2 pounds chicken breast, cut into strips

2 cups flour

1 cup milk

1 egg

Steak fries:
4 potatoes, cut into strips

3 tablespoons olive oil

Honey mustard dipping sauce:
2 tablespoons honey

2 tablespoons mustard

For the chicken tenders, scramble the egg and milk together. Dredge the chicken in flour, then dip into egg mixture. Bake according to your air fryer's instructions (about 15 minutes at 380°F, flipping once). For the steak fries, brush with oil, season as desired, and bake (about 12 minutes at 380°F, flipping once). Mix the honey and mustard, then dip and enjoy!

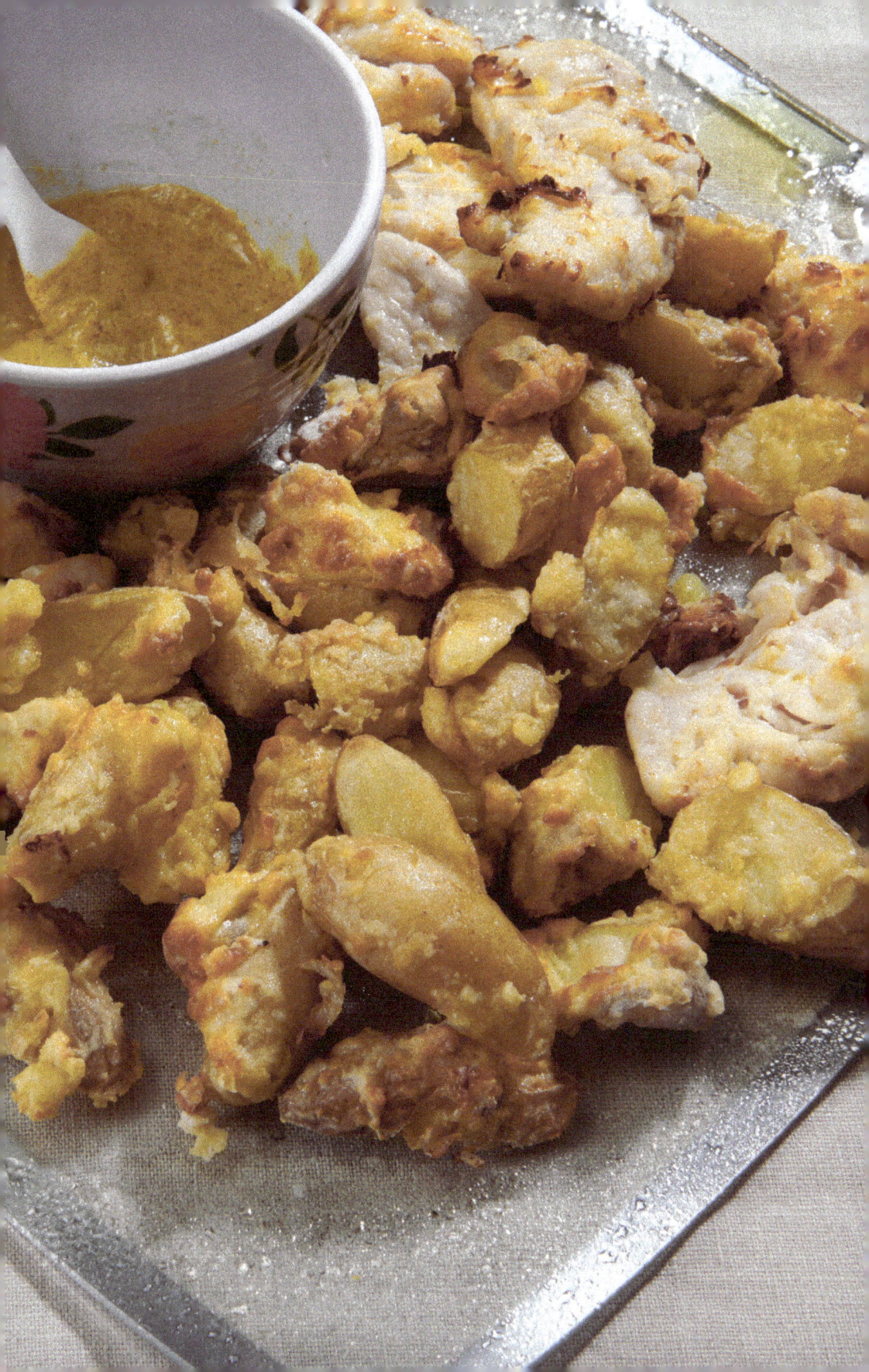

By carving out time and intention to do the things that make you feel fully alive, you are feeding yourself the most delicious meal you could ever make and enjoy. Feeling happy is the most satisfying and indulgent feeling of all. When you are happy, you lose all cravings for any other life than the one you are living right now. Plus, you naturally want to take care of yourself by eating well and exercising. It's a circle but not a vicious one. You will be surprised by the number of doors that open for you when you follow your heart, eat for fuel, and exercise for fun.

In the next chapter, I will explore ways to dress your best. This doesn't mean high fashion; it means dressing to fit your body type, using accessories wisely, learning to look in the mirror and like what you see, and finding the perfect outfit—in the store or in your own closet. I even give some ideas on how to lose a few pounds to fit into the perfect dress for a special event. Let's do this together!

INDULGE OR YOU'LL BULGE

RAG DOLL POSE

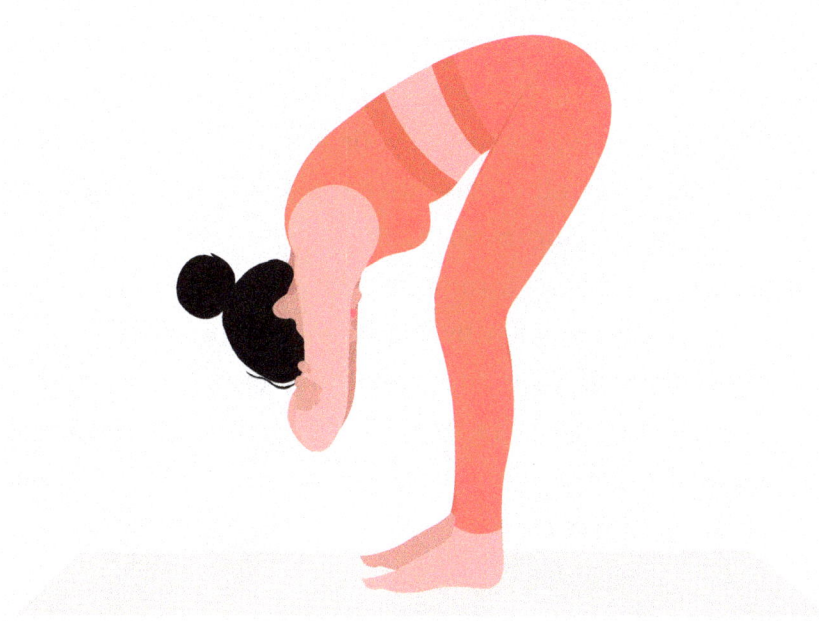

MOVE WITH MEANING

You've worked hard in the plank position, and now it's time to relax your body with the rag doll pose. As you feel your body flop downward, both your mind and body let loose. You are indulging in a moment of tranquility and self-love.

1. Start with your feet planted firmly on the ground.
2. Bend forward at your hips.
3. Become a rag doll and flop forward with your head hanging down between your arms.
4. Grasp your elbows with each hand and enjoy the stretch in your lower back.
5. Hang for about a minute and while you hang there, contemplate healthy indulgences you could incorporate into your life and think about how adding small indulgences to your days could help you stay on track with your diet goals and your overall personal happiness.

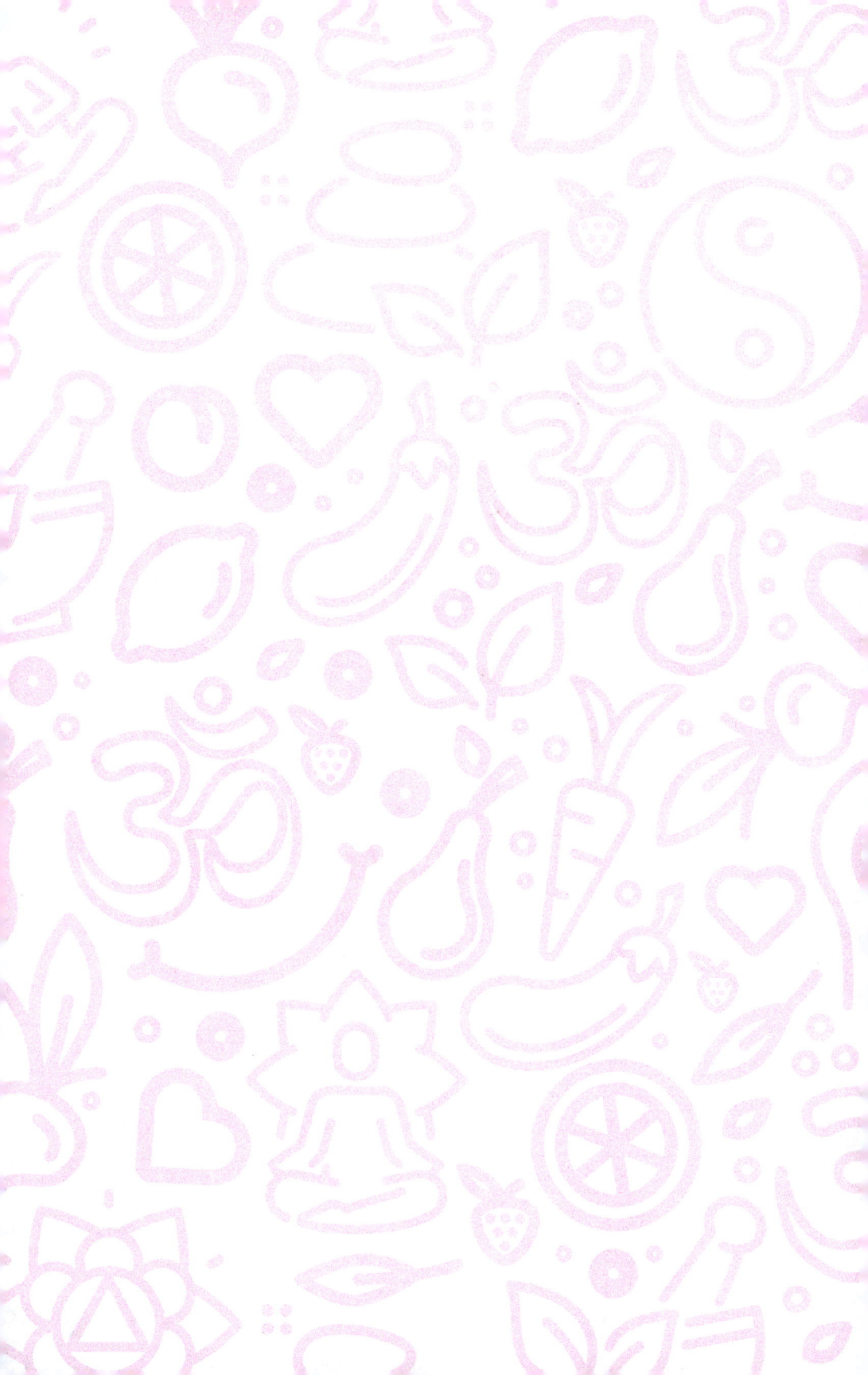

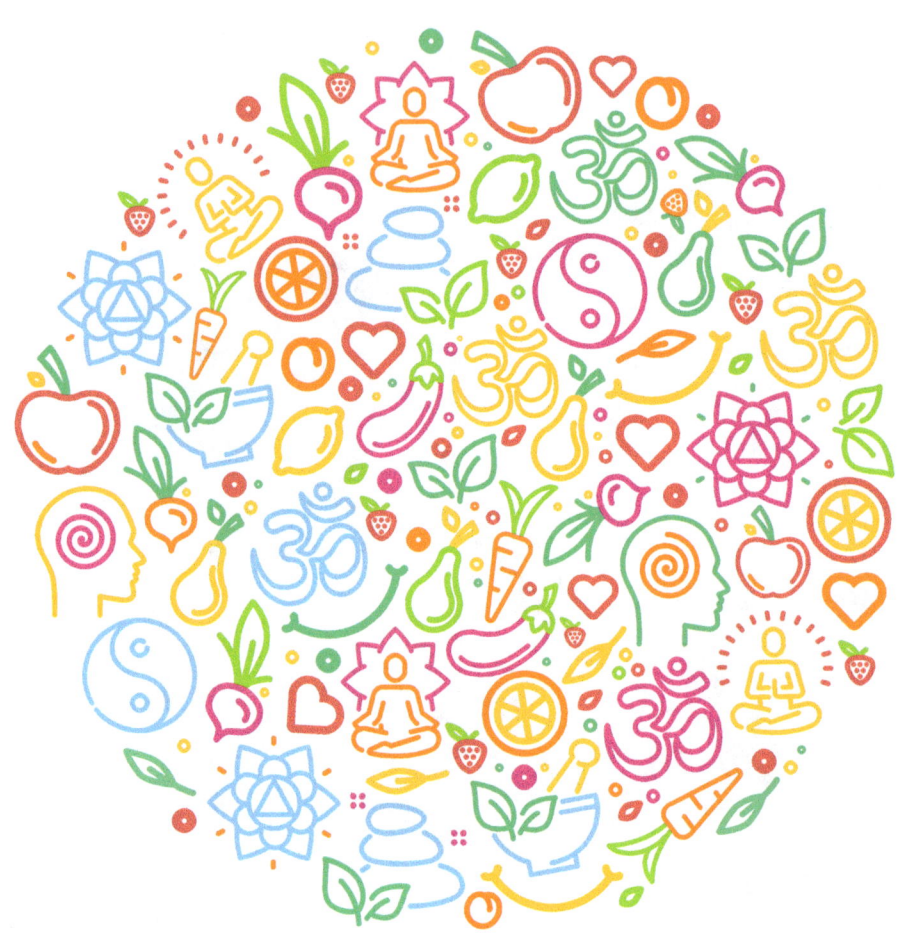

CHAPTER 10

Dress Your Best

Puttin' on the Ritz with Pudding Trifle

When I was a teenager, my mom enrolled my sister and me in a type of etiquette class. The idea of it was outlandish to us. We wondered why we were even doing it, but since we had each other, it simply became this hilarious thing that we had to do. Some of what the instructor said and made us do was ridiculous. Like the time she told us to never wear a miniskirt because knees are an ugly body part! Or when she instructed us to put Vaseline on our hands and cover them in white gloves every night so we would wake up with soft, succulent hands. (I'm not sure what the reasoning was. Possibly that a man couldn't resist holding our hands or that we looked like we never lifted a finger?)

She also taught us how to walk like a model and lectured us on how to stay thin. If we hadn't seen the class for what it was, we would have come out with a body complex. At the end of the class, she awarded a prize to the girls who made the most progress. My sister and I didn't win, and I was really upset. She said, "Maria and her sister came into the course with a good set of knowledge, so they didn't need much improvement." I was still mad! But it didn't stick. I knew deep down it was all nonsense.

Yet at their core, there was a nugget of truth in those etiquette lessons. It's this: when we outwardly present ourselves in a good light, we often feel better about ourselves. Have you ever gone to the grocery store in sweats, having not showered that day, and then bumped into someone you knew? There is a little sense of wanting to hide (at least for me—if not for you, I say, "You go, girl!"). It seems we all have our own limits of what we are comfortable with, and those limits change over time. The trick is finding what works for you; maybe it's no makeup or just lipstick or a dash of mascara and you are off, or maybe it's getting properly dressed and dolled up every time you step out the door. Whatever personal grooming and beauty habits suit you best—and make you feel good about yourself—are what you should do.

Beauty and grooming is a personal standard that you set for yourself, and it's just that: personal. It doesn't matter if it matches what society tells you is right or what habits your best friend has. That's a perk of getting older. As smart women who have mastered a lot of things in life, we have learned to come to ourselves for advice and guidance first, before going elsewhere. This inner confidence is extremely freeing. You've got it, so flaunt it!

Personally, I'm pretty versatile. If I am heading to an exercise class or out for a walk, all I need is to get in comfy workout gear, brush my teeth and hair, and head out the door. But my own personal rules say that if I am going to meet people out for a drink or dinner, then I should dress my best. That doesn't mean red-carpet ready every time, just something I feel good wearing. You don't have to look in the mirror every time you head out and say, "Well now, look who is the fairest of them all," but you should be able to look at yourself in the mirror and be happy with what you see.

As women, we can be our own worst critics. If you look in the mirror and focus on that one body part that you have always disliked and overlook your brand-spankin'-new outfit, what good is that? The next time you are tempted to judge yourself, force yourself to smile. Admire something you've always liked about yourself—your pretty face, the curve of your collarbone, your strong legs. Maybe even add a little jig and say to yourself, "I look good!" If you do it often enough, you will start to believe it. And you should!

The better you look, the better you feel.

Let's talk clothes. For me, putting together outfits is a creative act, much like cooking. I gather this ingredient—a pair of black slim-cut jeans—and mix it with another ingredient—a beautiful blouse—then add a topping of classic jewelry and secret ingredients of a hip belt and ankle boots, and voilà!

While my Nana, my maternal grandmother, shared her cooking wisdom with me, my paternal grandmother's gift was teaching me how to shop. Her biggest message was "Skip the bargain bin! Let's go full cost." She couldn't be bothered with sales and sifting through racks and racks of clothing that didn't make other women's first cut. It's a great concept because the hidden message is "Value yourself." Of course we can't always break the bank for clothing, but once in a while it's important to treat yourself with something that feels perfect.

When you shop, go with a plan in mind. If you walk into a boutique starry eyed with nothing but a credit card and hours to use it, you are going to end up buying a few items you will likely never wear. Instead, think about that beautiful blouse that is hanging in your closet and shop for a way to dress it up, like with black slacks or a long black skirt.

Also, flip through fashion magazines now and then. It helps you step out of a rut and consider a new look. It sparks an awareness about what colors you like and what is trending. (Not that you have to honor that! I will never buy a pair of ripped jeans, for example. I leave those for my girls to buy.) You can't take fashion advice from the red carpet, but it's fun to see how people put outfits together and glean a few tricks that resonate. Also, pay attention to the mannequins in the store. What are they rockin' that works?

Even though I often like to shop alone because I find clothes to be such a personal thing, it helps to bring a trusted girlfriend or a family member along to get a second opinion. Only bring someone you know will be honest. I love the smooth lines of Ralph Lauren, but with my short stature his pants would go up to my chin! Even if your friend says you look good in something, check in with yourself while alone in the dressing room. Clothes are your form of personal expression. If what you put on doesn't make you feel good, don't get it, no matter how hard someone tries to persuade you.

When in doubt on whether to buy something or not, ask yourself if it is something you'd wear to a casual gathering with friends. If the answer is yes, you are more likely to wear it, so buy it! So many events are smart casual these days. And no matter what, try the outfit on rather than eyeballing it in a rush. I get it that going in the dressing room at this age isn't always fun, but it's best to make yourself do it. It's not worth the effort to return it later.

We have to talk about shoes. I love shoes. If you are going to blow your budget on anything, do it on shoes. I used to wear stilettos, but they ruined my feet. Now it's platforms for me all the way. Even then, if I am going dancing, I will put ballet flats in my purse for later. Being the wise, older woman that I am, I always put comfort above style, every time.

Shopping shouldn't be a hassle. Once it starts feeling less like fun and more like work, quit. You want it to give you a lift and be enjoyable. It should be like eating a yummy dessert like my quick Pudding Trifle. If the event you're dressing for is a potluck, bring it along!

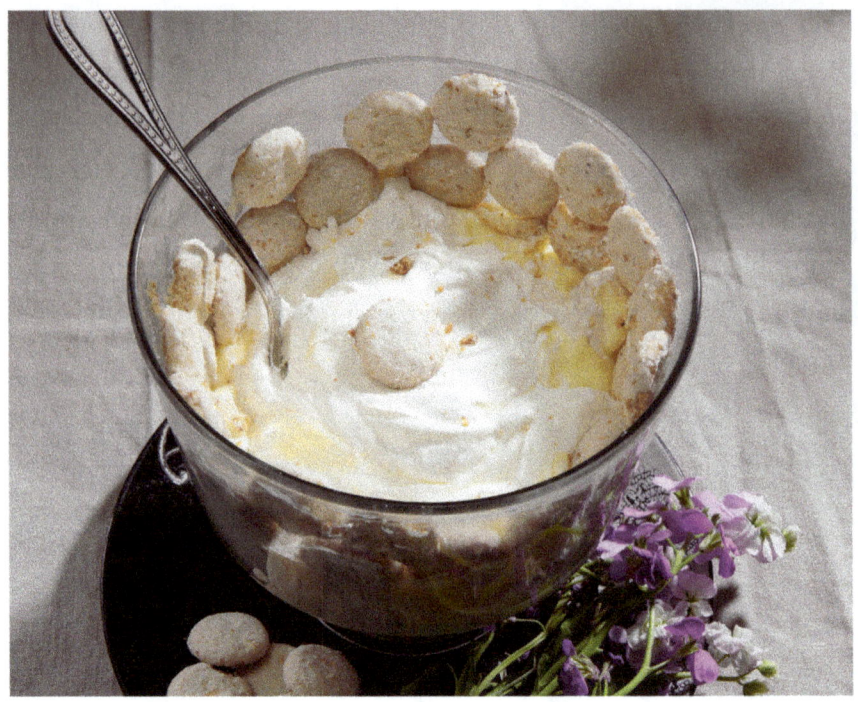

Pudding Trifle

> 2 (8-ounce) packages vanilla pudding
> 1 box lemon or lime powdered sugar cookies (store-bought)
> 1 (8-ounce) tub nondairy whipped topping

Pour pudding in a large bowl. Spread layer of whipped topping. Top with cookies.

Of course, there are times when you need a fancy outfit, and that demands throwing caution to the wind (along with your pocketbook) and finding something fabulous. In reality, you don't have to spend a lot. I recently bought two dresses for an event, and I posted on

Instagram asking which outfit people liked better. Guess what? The majority chose the inexpensive outfit I bought at a chain store! It's like wine: the most expensive bottle doesn't always taste the best. That says something about how dressing your best can be more about how an item hangs on you rather than the price tag itself. Clothing has to fit your shape, your style, and your coloring.

In fact, I often start shopping in my closet. I walk in as if I'm in a boutique and I see what items I still gaze at fondly. The ones that I imagine feeling good out in public in, I keep. The rest I weed out and give to charity. It's these items that help me create my shopping list. Sometimes all that's on my shopping list is the perfect scarf, a stylish belt, or a fancy hair piece to dress up my favorite cream dress.

An accessory can make an outfit. When you start in your closet first, you can create a new outfit for less than a hundred dollars. Sometimes it helps to organize your closet by outfits rather than by items (shirt, slacks, etc.), including accessories. Or consider organizing by seasons. I believe your closet should be a rainbow of colors. Also, don't forget to do spring cleaning. Spring is my favorite season. It's a time for rejuvenation, so rejuvenate your closet and your life. With less clutter, you will be able to more easily contrive a perfect outfit from what's hanging right in front of you.

For a special event, I often have a plan A and plan B outfit, and sometimes a C and D! And there are many times I have gone with plan D. That's because when the event comes, your mood might not fit your dress, or you feel bloated and you are not sure you want to wear something formfitting. Or your feet hurt, so you decide to go with the outfit that matches your most comfy shoes.

GIVE BLOAT THE BOOT

Bloating is unpleasant. It doesn't feel good, and it doesn't look good, but it happens to all of us. For those of us in menopause, it's even more common because fluctuating hormone levels influence every aspect of how our bodies function, including digestion. Try these dietary and exercise changes to help give bloat the boot:

- If you want to fit into your favorite little black dress for an event, avoid cruciferous vegetables like broccoli, cauliflower, and Brussels sprouts a few days beforehand. They are slow to digest, which can lead to gassy bloat.[17]
- We all know that beans and legumes create gassiness. Avoid them or soak them well. To lessen their negative effects, soak them in water for eight to twelve hours prior to cooking. Cooking them in a pressure cooker may help further break down their gas-causing compounds.
- Alliums such as onions, garlic, and shallots are also known gas producers, so use them in moderation. Cooking them until they're very soft and tender also helps.
- Here's one more reason to reduce your sugar intake. Sugar exacerbates digestive problems by feeding the bad bacteria in our guts. Even some

---

17 Cleveland Clinic Health Essentials, "15 Foods That Can Cause Bloating," accessed August 20, 2022, https://health.clevelandclinic.org/foods-that-cause-bloating.

fruits that are high in sugar, like pineapple, can cause bloating.
- Drink up! Staying well hydrated can aid in reducing bloating by keeping things moving through your gut.
- Too much salt can cause you to retain water and bloat. Lessening your salt intake can reduce bloating by about a quarter.[18]
- Movement helps to reduce bloating by eliminating gas that has built up in the digestive tract.

Just like with cooking a special meal, dressing well takes quality time. Don't skimp on how much time you take to get ready for an event or rush through getting dressed, doing your hair, and prepping your makeup. You are practicing self-care when you give yourself the time you need to get ready so that you can feel great walking out the door. How is that a bad way to spend your time? The trick is looking like you spent five minutes when you really spent five hours! Remember, your outer appearance is the first impression you make, so make it a good one—make it one that says, "This is who I am, world! Watch out! Here I come."

The same goes for your hairstyle. Pick a style that complements the shape of your face. For example, textured, layered hair is good for women with round faces because it draws the eye away from the jawline. If you have a long face, try a medium-length curly style that

---

18   Harvard Health Publishing, "Problems with Bloating? Watch Your Sodium Intake," accessed August 23, 2022, https://www.health.harvard.edu/staying-healthy/problems-with-bloating-watch-your-sodium-intake.

gives your face the illusion of extra width. If you have a hairdresser you like, stick with them. Don't stray even if you get a cut that you don't love. By now they know you and your hair, so at your next appointment simply be a little more assertive about what you want.

It's easy to think a new stylist or makeup artist can give you a better look, but that's not usually the case. However, if you are sporting the same hairstyle that you had in college, go out right now and change it! After all, your face isn't the same shape it was in the '80s. At least try something new for a while. You can always go back to your old cut.

Speaking of hair, it's okay to dye your hair to keep the natural color you were born with (or explore a new, exciting one), and it's okay to let your gray hair make a strong, beautiful statement, just as long as it's an intentional choice and one that fits you. Mostly, don't get bored with your look. Boredom is the kiss of death.

And nails? I say, give up trying to do them at home and go to the salon. The last time I tried to paint my toenails, it looked like a child who painted outside of the lines. Let's face it: our eyesight is going to keep getting worse. After all, part of aging is accepting our limitations!

Another way I feed both my outer and inner beauty is caring for my aging skin. I'm not one to go for a ton of procedures to make my face appear younger than my natural age, but I do enjoy taking good care of it. I'm growing older, and that's okay. Instead of denying my age, I accept and enjoy my age with grace, taking with me the good stuff and leaving behind the bad. This approach is like a yoga meditation, where you focus on what is good in your life and weed out the rest. I live in the moment, right smack in my current age.

In Italy, women are perceived differently. You are less likely to see women having a midlife crisis in Italy. Women in their eighties and nineties wear bikinis at the beach. Isn't that wonderful? As Americans, we have to ask ourselves, "What are we ashamed of?" Let's take a lesson from these European women and love ourselves exactly how we are. Let's change our perspective on the aging process. Let's respect ourselves and other women as we grow older.

At the same time, we want to look our best to feel our best. European women find a nice balance with this in their lives. They accept their bodies but still value outward beauty. If you are not feeling good about who you are mentally or physically, you are less likely to commit to wellness. To rejuvenate your face, try my six tips. Of course, consult with your dermatologist to see if my regimen is right for you.

MARIA'S SIX HELPFUL TIPS FOR A BEAUTIFUL FACE

1. **Protect against the sun.** Feeling the sun on your face is glorious, but in your fifties, you have to be diligent with sunscreen. Use SPF 50 and get in the habit of putting it on in the morning and reapplying it throughout the day. Buy a cute summer hat and don't forget to pack it for outdoor events.
2. **Drink water with lemon.** Stay hydrated to keep your complexion smooth.
3. **Limit alcohol, caffeine, and sugar.** Too much clogs your pores, and the excess is reflected in the texture and pallor of your skin.
4. **The biggie: get seven to nine hours of sleep a night!** Sleep is extra important as we age to counter stress and recharge. If you are tired, your face will show it.

5. **Make homemade facials.** Find a recipe with avocado, banana, or honey; those are my favorites, but experiment on your own. Fruit of the earth is always good.
6. **Don't be afraid to watch makeup tutorials.** We all need a little help learning how to apply makeup that works best with our personal look. Who knows? You might discover that more than one look agrees with you.

Let's talk about losing a few pounds to fit into a special dress for an event. While I don't approve of crash dieting, I do appreciate goal-oriented dieting. If you have an upcoming event for which you want to look fabulous—say, a nephew's wedding, your daughter's graduation, or your thirtieth high school reunion—and you want to feel good about yourself, go ahead and make a plan to lose five pounds the month before, but no more.

The goal isn't to change your entire body shape, just to lose a few pounds so the dress fits well. Mostly, you do it for yourself as a confidence boost. After all, you have an established weight-management plan that helps you keep your weight in the same ballpark. When you want to lose a little weight, I recommend my temporary steady-as-she-goes diet.

MARIA'S STEADY-AS-SHE-GOES DIET

If you want to lose those five pesky pounds, try my simple diet for a few weeks. It provides easy, low-cal meal options. If you stick to this for a week, I bet you lose a pound or two. Feel free to switch up these meals, like having dinner for breakfast or breakfast for lunch to suit your taste. A wise person once said, "Don't be a slave to the clock!"

Breakfast Options

A. Half of a hollowed-out bagel with ricotta cheese

B. Scrambled egg with tomato, herbs, and a dollop of ricotta cheese

Lunch Options

A. Salad consisting of lettuce, veggies of choice, and three ounces of protein (chicken, turkey, hard-boiled egg, tuna, tofu) and topped with a few teaspoons of nuts/seeds and a sprinkle of shredded cheese (for dressing, make a simple balsamic dressing with a quarter cup of olive oil, a splash of balsamic vinegar, and a dash of sea salt)

B. Tomato soup (if you don't have a can of soup, make your own by combining a can of tomatoes with a can of chicken broth and boiling it) topped with a sprinkle of cheese

Dinner Options

A. Fish or poultry with a small side of pasta, potato, brown rice, or quinoa and a vegetable of choice

B. A low-cal dinner from this book or from my website at officialmariasabando.com (on occasion, have one alcoholic drink or a little dessert like a small scoop of ice cream or a few squares of chocolate)

Snacks

You know I like my snacks! At your hungriest part of the day, have one snack. This can be a handful of nuts, one cup of bone broth, a piece of fruit, or a low-cal protein bar.

Drink a lot of water and herbal tea, and don't forget to exercise! Three to four times a week works for me. Good luck!

My Pepper Steak, minus the side of bread, is a tasty, low-cal dinner that you can have while dieting. The portion below is meant to be shared. It's bound to leave you satisfied.

Pepper Steak

- 1½ pounds sirloin or filet mignon
- 2 peppers, sliced julienne style (cut thin, like matchsticks)
- 3 teaspoons olive oil
- 1 teaspoon favorite hot sauce

Warm oil in pan. Add meat and peppers. Stir and sear the meat until it is medium rare or a desired redness. Mix in hot sauce.

As you gain momentum with your temporary diet, try on the dress to see how far you have to go. Resist the urge to chastise yourself or speed up the weight-loss process. Instead, look for small changes, like how it feels slightly looser in your hips. If you lose a single pound, celebrate! I find losing even a little weight is incredibly motivating and helps

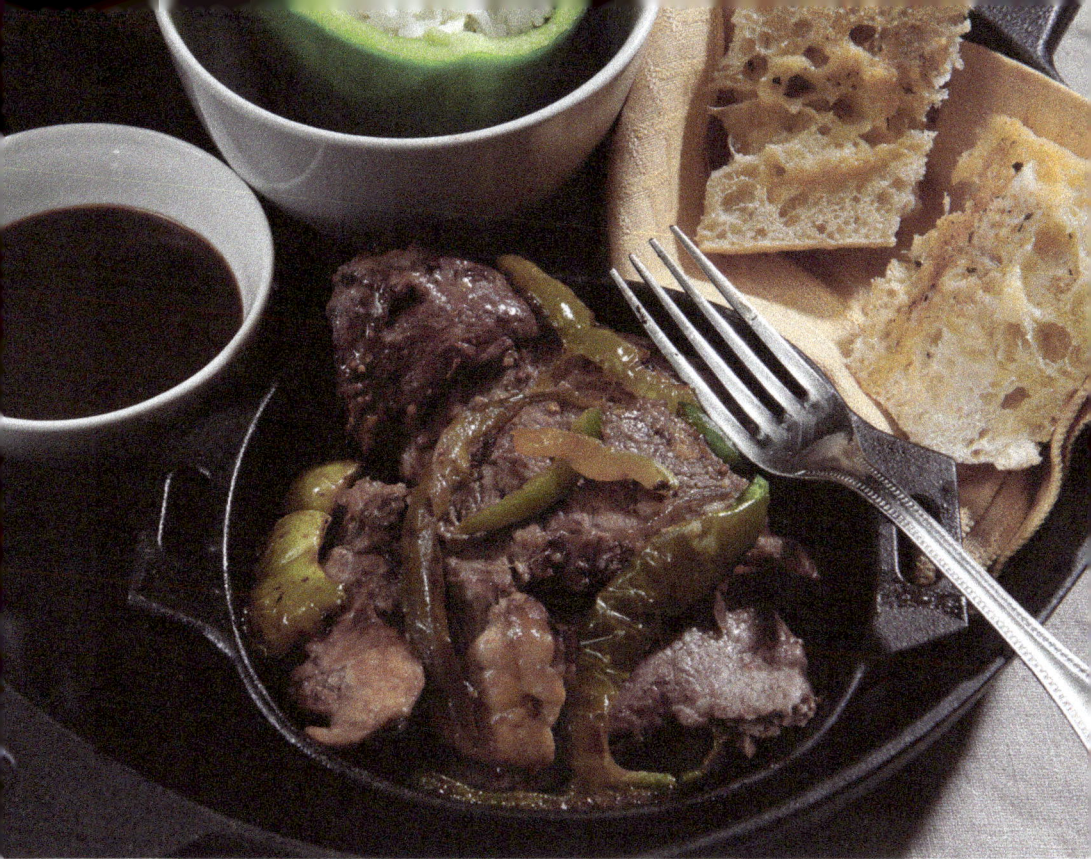

me stick to my diet. Losing weight slowly and steadily is healthier and often comes with lifestyle changes that have sticking power for keeping the pounds off. Keep your eye on the prize—hey, I didn't say it would be a cakewalk (no cake until the actual event)! Besides, all that healthy food is going to make your skin glow!

In the next chapter, we'll dive into party planning with lots of ideas on how to throw a healthy, fun event. I answer questions like "When should I cater, and when should I cook?" "What fun themes really entice guests?" and other questions you maybe don't even know that you are dying to ask. Get ready! Let's go!

LOVING LIFE AT 50+

CHAIR SQUAT

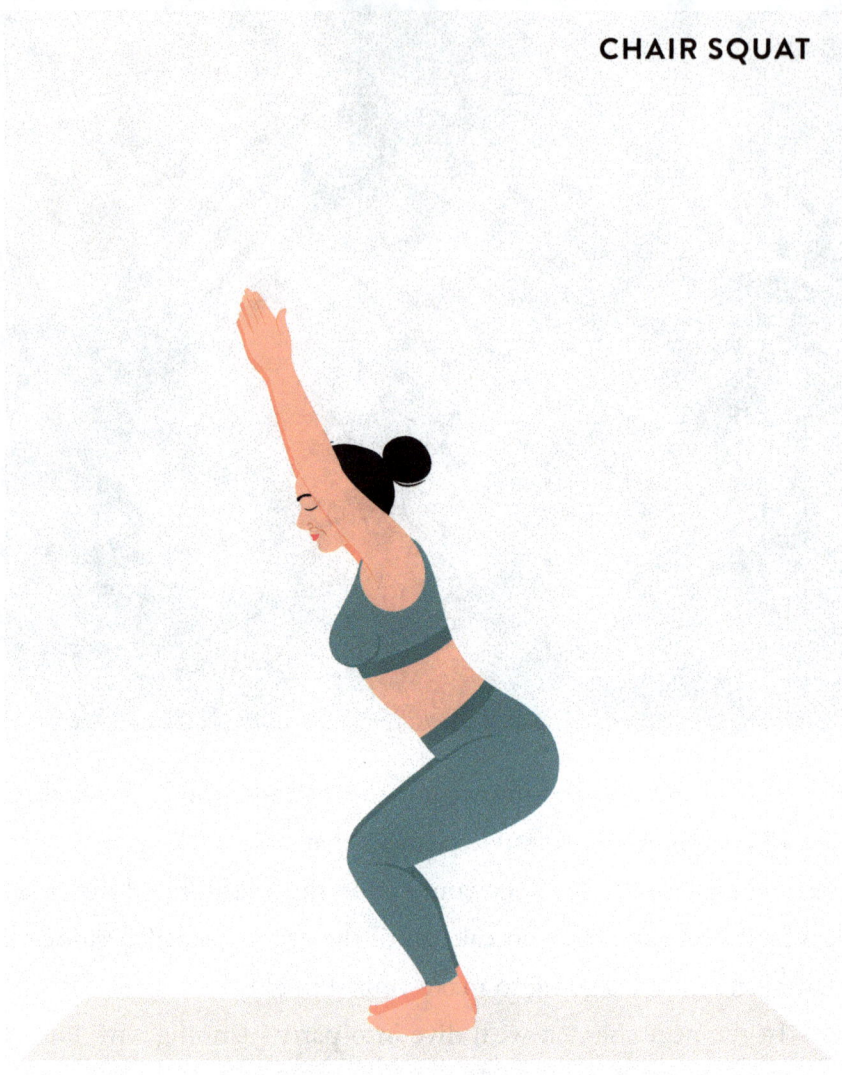

MOVE WITH MEANING

If you are going to look great in your favorite dress, you want your backside to be nicely shaped. That's where the chair squat comes in. It's a harder exercise than flow yoga, but it's great to do as part of a yoga session or even just a few times throughout the day. It really shapes your glutes, quads, and hamstrings. The chair squat is also good for improving your balance and overall strength. So rise up out of your rag doll pose and get ready to work.

1. For the chair squat, you can use an actual chair or an invisible one.
2. Stand with your back to the chair, keeping your chest raised and your spine in a straight position.
3. Put your arms high over your head, parallel to each other.
4. Squat down to where you can feel the chair with your bottom. Just tap it—don't sit on it.
5. Squeeze your glutes tight and push your hips forward.
6. Hold the pose for as long as you can, starting with ten seconds. Repeat five times, resting in between.

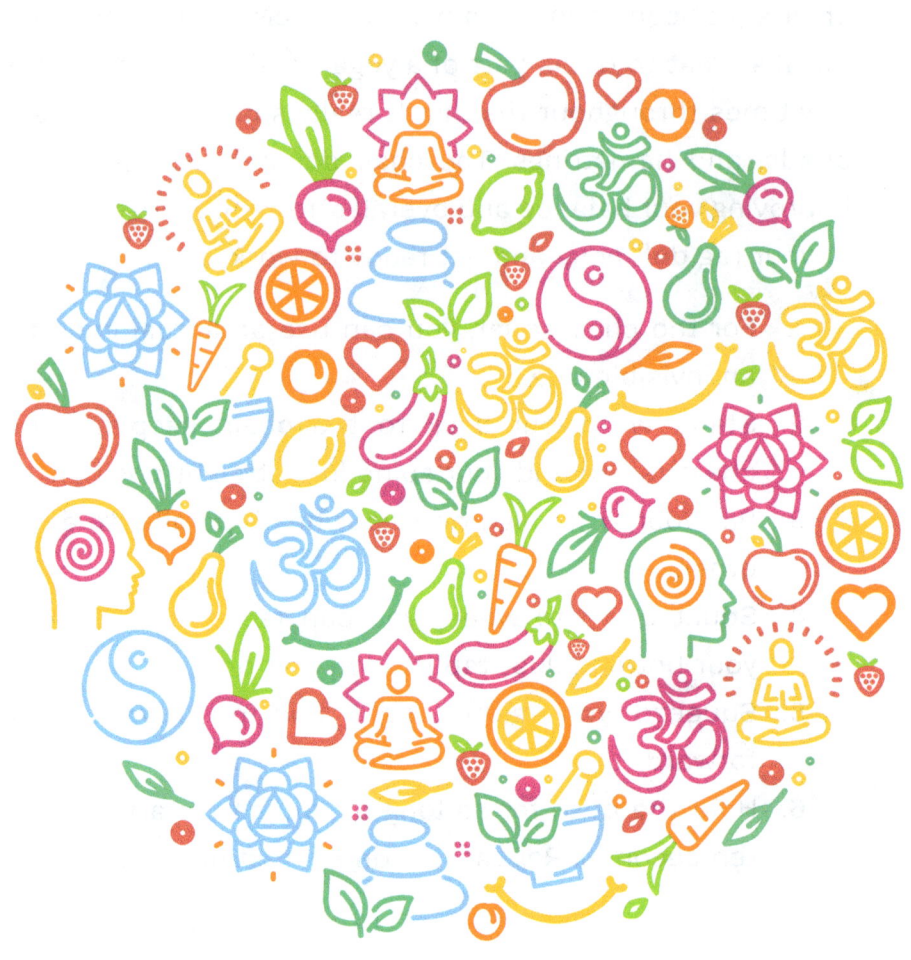

CHAPTER 11

Party for Health!
Get Together over a Tasty Taco Bar

My friends know that I get easily bored and I like to throw fun, crazy parties. While I like to host themed parties that are centered around yoga, makeovers, and fashion, some of the best parties that I have are spontaneous. They're more girls' nights than actual parties. This summer, I've had girls come over for some light exercise followed by a swim and a drink by the pool, where we gab and gossip. We women need to get together regularly to talk and vent. It is almost like we are teenagers again. Now that my youngest daughter is off to college, I have more time for both planned theme parties and girls' nights out.

To kick it off, I'm hosting a fall party for a friend. It's really just an excuse for us to come together and dish, shop, and adorn ourselves. What's fun about having a social gathering at your home is that you can control the food, drinks, and activities. Even for spontaneous gatherings, I have a themed drink and snacks. My friends appreciate my hospitality, and they think I am doing them a favor, but really, they are doing me the favor! As I get older, I cherish my friendships more and more. We have to make time for fun, which, along with healthy food and good exercise, keeps us young.

Partying with family and friends is essential to happy living: food tastes better when it's enjoyed with others. I love prepping for parties. It gets my adrenaline going as I run around the kitchen cooking and plating food, putting the last touches on my makeup, and making sure the house is presentable. It's work, but it's good work. In fact, sometimes at the end of a night of entertaining, I have the same feeling as I do after taking a cardio class—happily spent.

While you might think that hosting parties and always being around food would make you gain weight, I find the opposite to be true. I actually lose weight during the holidays because of all the running around during preparation. It's also good for our brains as we age. Party planning and hosting sharpens your mind and your skills. You have to multitask with cooking, socializing, and making sure your guests are comfortable. With that said, you don't want to feel stressed or exhausted from the preparation. Plan ahead so that you have enough time to feel relaxed while getting ready. That way, you will feel refreshed when you come down to the kitchen and simply pull out the appetizers that are all set to go.

If you want to throw a party and you don't know where to begin, start with a theme. Themes make it easier to pick the menu and start planning. You don't have to go crazy. If it is more of a loose get-together, just have a themed drink and some easy, ready-made appetizers to serve. A signature drink shows that you care enough about your guests that you wanted to plan and make it fun. It sets the mood for a good time. One of my favorite signature drinks is a Bellini. It's an Italian cocktail made with prosecco and peach puree, with a slice of peach as a garnish. Remember to chill the champagne flutes beforehand. Yum! Or make a signature dessert instead, like my Berry Salad that's featured in chapter 6, which is super easy and celebratory. Bring out the Martha Stewart in you, because she's in there!

> **There is no single recipe for success. But there is one essential ingredient: passion.**
> —Martha Stewart

For my girlfriends, sometimes I plan a yoga party followed by drinks and healthy snacks. Yoga parties are great because I get to share my skills with others. I have earned two hundred hours toward the four hundred hours that I need to gain my certification, so I get more practice teaching, and they get the benefit of a great yoga class. Lately, I've been into sculpt yoga, where you introduce weights into the yoga session. What's great is that teaching yoga classes keeps me exercising regularly, so I can meet my own fitness goals. Consider your own skills and how you could share them with others in a fun way. When you teach something to someone, it feels good.

At times, I have thrown a makeover party, where I bring in a talented makeup artist to give us all ideas on enhancing our looks and enjoying the change we see in each other. Another fun idea is a craft party. When I'm feeling creative, I'll go to the craft store and get supplies for a unique project. I've made cell phone carrier cases, command stations to organize schedules, mason suggestion jars, and more. Are you in a book club? The next time your group gets together, offer to host and theme the party to the book. Make food and drinks that the characters in the book enjoyed (or you think they would enjoy based on their personalities). Suggest that everyone wear one item that speaks of the time or tone of the book—say, a flouncy hat or a vintage hairpin if you are reading *Pride and Prejudice*. You can even make up trivia questions related to the book to get the discussion going. My friends know I love my themed parties. They keep me from getting bored.

When considering food to serve, you don't want a strictly themed party—like vegan food only. Rather, make items that are sure to please the whole crowd, such as my Varied Taco Bar, which has something for everyone.

Varied Taco Bar

> Taco shells
> 1 pound shrimp
> Hummus (store-bought)
> Green and red pepper, sliced

Depending on how many tacos you need, steam shrimp, then salt and drizzle with olive oil. Warm the taco shells. Fill some shells with shrimp and other shells with hummus. Top with pepper slices. Serve with store-bought salsa and guacamole on the side.

If you have several friends who are vegan or vegetarian, it will mean a lot to them to have a special dish that they can enjoy when they come to your house for a party. They will know that you put in the extra effort to please them, and that feels good. I suggest my Tofu Soup. It's healthy and delicious, and it won't cause anyone to break their weight-management diets.

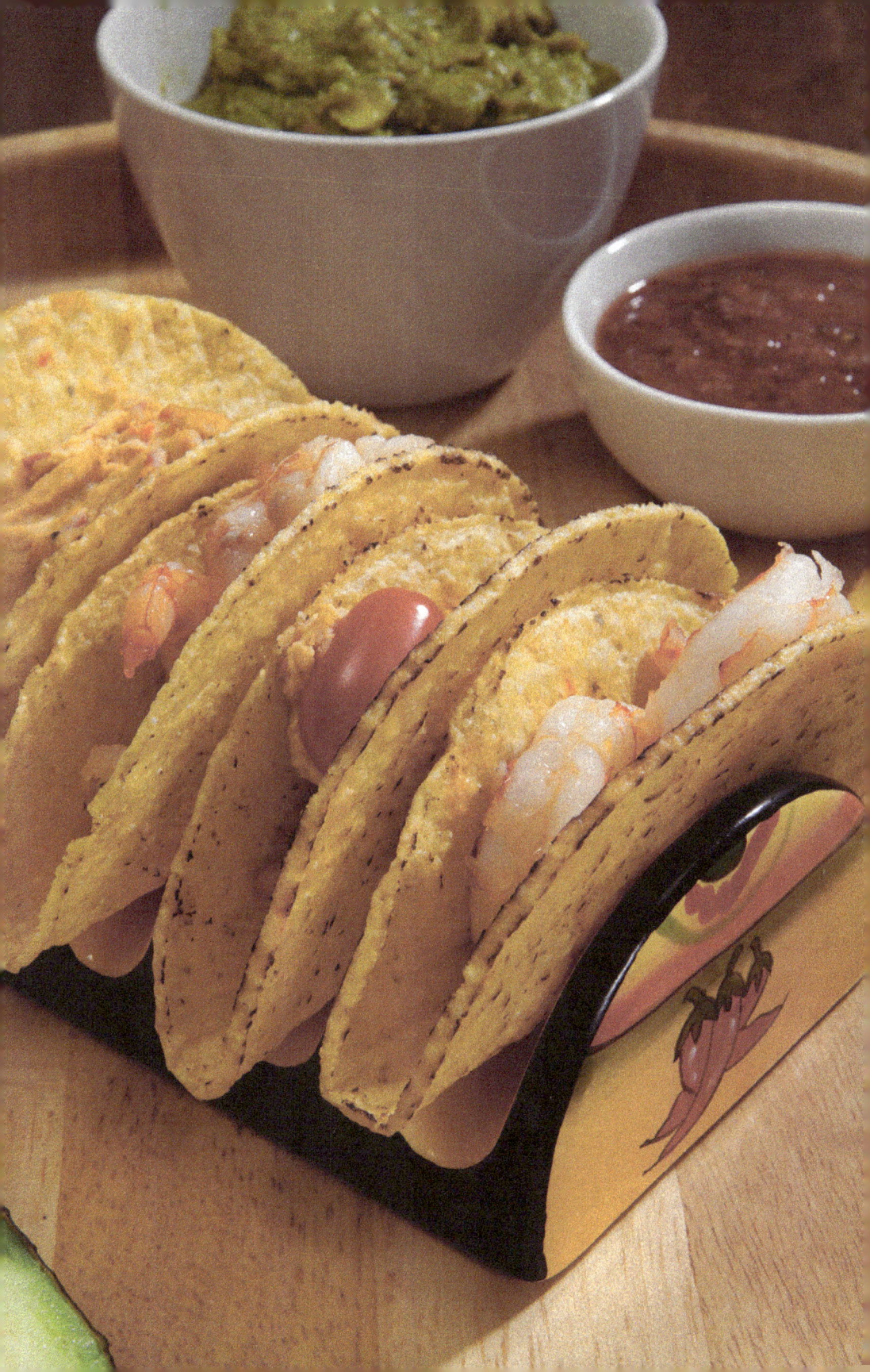

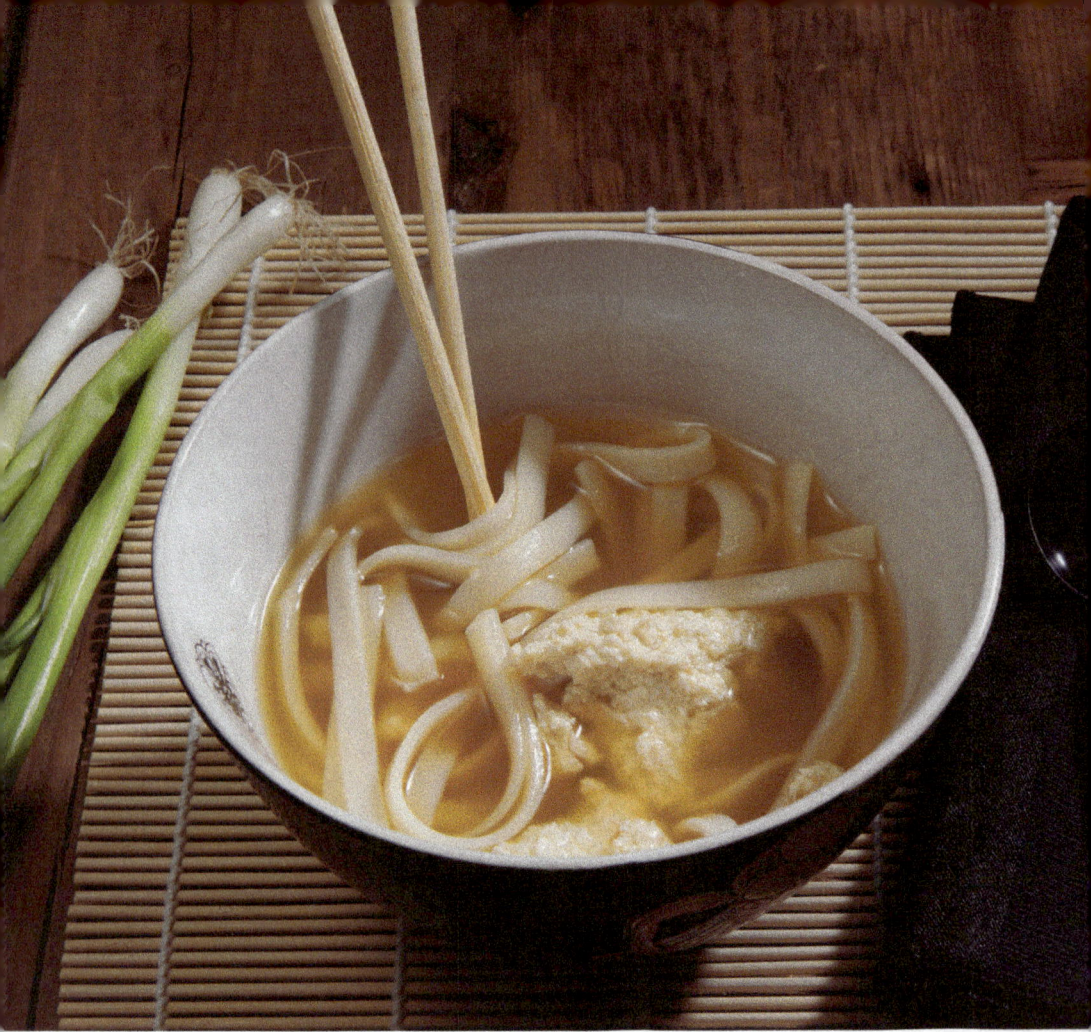

Tofu Soup

- 1 tablespoon sesame oil
- 1 tablespoon lite soy sauce
- ½ box brown rice noodles
- 1 box vegetable broth
- 1 cup firm tofu

Boil all ingredients over medium heat. Lower heat; cover. Allow to simmer for 15 minutes.

As a child, I remember family barbecues where we would all sit on the screened-in porch and visit. Sometimes we had clambakes with steamers. A family memory that we laugh about is how my mother would make me wear a life jacket in the baby pool! Another, more recent funny memory was a time when we were having a party at the Jersey Shore and my husband's cousin parked his van in a part of the parking lot that was restricted by cones. We were at the beach having fun when we noticed his van sinking down in the sand. He was so embarrassed that he wanted to jump in the bay and swim out into the ocean! Families are crazy, so enjoy the chaotic, joyous, loving mess that is your family.

When hosting a large, important event, like your best friend's fiftieth birthday party or your daughter's college graduation party, consider having it catered. What's most important during these special family or friend events is that you get to be undistracted and present to soak in the special moment. You want to be relaxed and indulge in good conversations and fun activities without the worry of wondering whether or not an appetizer plate needs to be replenished or if your great-aunt needs her sherry refilled. The degree of how meaningful the event is for me is my litmus test for whether or not I will have it catered. If it means a lot to me to attend without interruptions or worry, I have the event catered.

When planning a big event, start by creating your guest list. This will help you determine the theme. If the crowd will include both adults and children, it's best to have some fun activities. Set up cornhole, boccie ball, and other yard games. Consider the dietary restrictions of your guests. Also, have some kid-friendly foods. Don't forget to make or buy special nonalcoholic drinks for the kids and nondrinkers. Choose a wide variety of foods to be catered or homemade, from healthy salads for your vegetarian friends to chicken skewers for the carnivores in your crowd. I like to serve tasty Antipasti for special family gatherings.

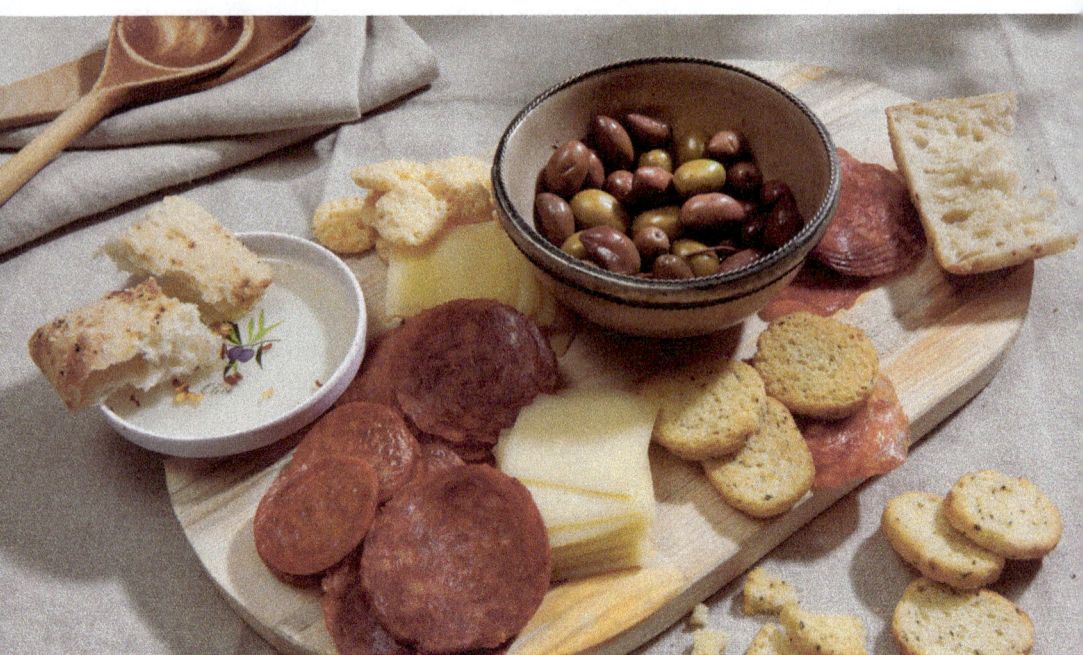

Antipasti

⅛ pound salami
⅛ pound pepperoni
¼ pound sliced provolone cheese
1 cup assorted olives
Italian rolls
¼ cup olive oil with chili flakes for dipping

Arrange all meats and cheeses on a wooden board. Place olives in a bowl in the center of the tray. Place bread or crackers on one side of the board and dipping oil on the opposite side.

Before the big event, ask for help. Recruit a friend to come early to wash the glasses or polish the silverware and arrange it nicely. If it is a fancy event, like a groom's dinner or bridal party, get a tent and ask the caterers to secure linens.

Start all this special party planning with a budget. Determine the maximum you would like to spend and don't stray too far. It's easy to get carried away, but you don't have to. Good food, good company, and a few special touches, like flowers and candles on the tables, and a table with photos honoring the guest of honor, are enough. Start planning well in advance to make sure the caterer is available and you have plenty of time to mull over special party touches. I always make an elaborate list of what I need to do for the party, which I often do not follow, due to my penchant for creativity. But that's okay: there's something to say for updating your plans as you go along. The days leading up to the event, treat yourself. Go to the salon and have your hair and nails done, or buy a new dress. After all, the lady of the house is stepping out for the night!

Let's talk about holidays. A great time to celebrate family is during the holidays. These moments in time are designed to make us set down our work, slow down, and just be together. We all have holiday traditions with family and friends. Our Christmas Eve celebration is special, because it morphs my Italian heritage with my husband's Ecuadorean roots. The champagne is always flowing, and the appetizers always include ceviche from my husband's side (look for his delicious recipe in the next chapter) and Antipasti (see above) and Red Sangria from my Italian side.

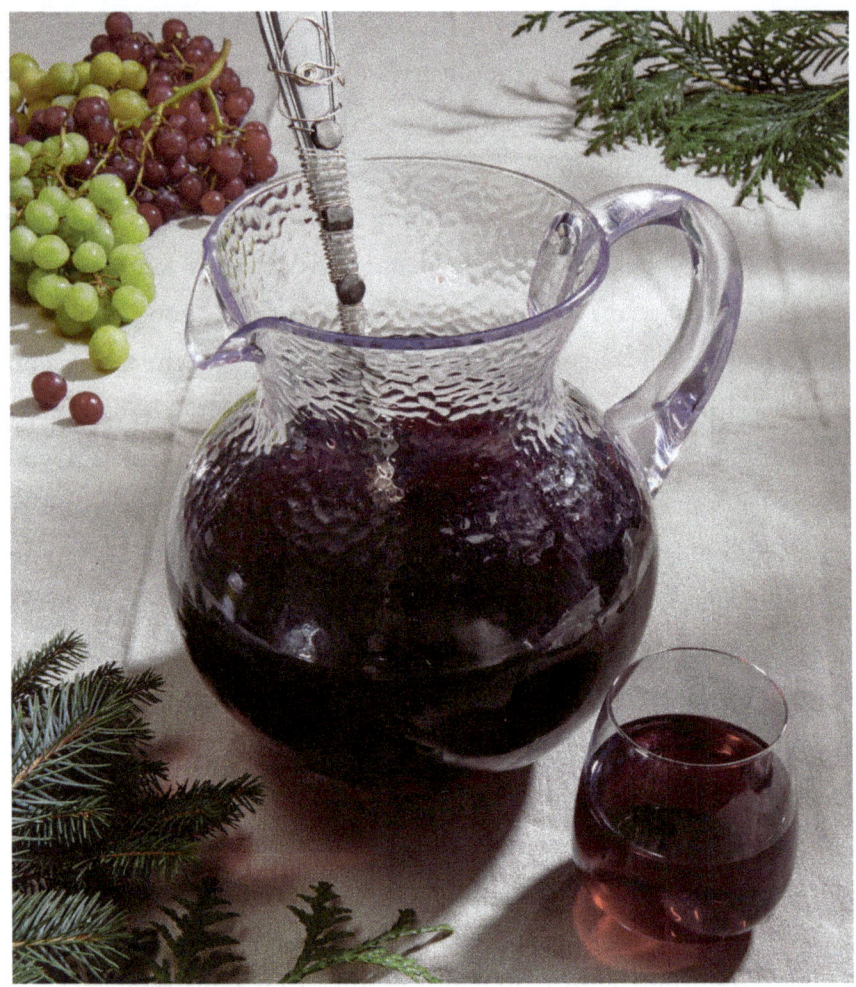

Red Sangria

1 large bottle of red sangria
1 cup green grapes
1 cup red grapes
1 cup maraschino cherries
2 cups ice

Mix all ingredients in a large pitcher with a long spoon.

What holiday recipes did your family pass down through the years? It's important to keep traditions alive, and food is a great way to do that. It's comforting to experience the same foods every year at the holidays, and it brings families closer together, helping to solidify family bonds.

For holiday celebrations, I go all out with decorations and party favors. Why not? It's a reason to get colorful and festive. I like to provide little gifts for my guests. At Easter, I make individual small baskets with goodies and set them at each plate setting. In my family, Easter is a cherished holiday. I keep it fun with my Carrot Muffins.

Carrot Muffins

- ¼ cup maple syrup
- ¼ cup unsweetened applesauce
- 2 eggs, beaten
- ¼ cup dairy or almond milk
- ½ teaspoon vanilla
- 1 cup whole wheat flour
- ¼ teaspoon baking powder
- ¼ teaspoon salt
- ½ cup chopped carrots
- ⅓ cup chopped walnuts
- ¼ cup confectioners' sugar

Spray the muffin tin with cooking spray. Mix syrup, applesauce, eggs, almond milk, and vanilla in a large bowl. In a separate bowl, combine flour, baking powder, and salt. Add dry mixture to wet and mix well. Add chopped carrots and stir lightly. Fill muffin cups with ½ cup batter per cup. Sprinkle nuts over each muffin. Bake at 350°F for 20 minutes. Cool for 10 minutes. Remove from tin with a plastic fork and sprinkle with confectioners' sugar. If desired, frost to create cupcakes. Makes 12 muffins.

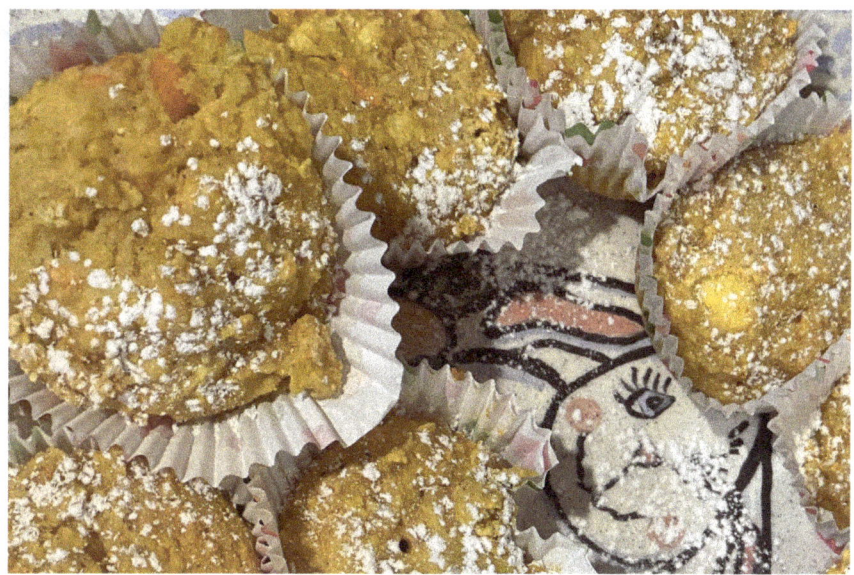

There's one Christmas tradition I didn't keep up with from my heritage. It was simply too time-consuming—making *struffoli*, Italian honey balls. As a child, I remember the Italian mothers all getting together and patiently rolling out balls of dough, which would then be made into this glorious tower of sticky goodness.

We would also attend the Feast of San Gennaro in the fall, which has been going on for nearly one hundred years in Little Italy in New York, New York. Talk about traditions! In Little Italy, the food was insanely good, from fritto misto—crispy, light fried shrimp, calamari, and zucchini—to delectable pastries and cannoli. One year I literally ate the brains of an animal, considered by some a delicacy. (I never said I was a vegetarian!)

Christmas at our house, and maybe yours, always includes a well-stocked cookie tray. I make almond balls, sugar cookies, cookie loaves, etc. etc. It's a must to have special drinks for the holidays. For Christmas, I like to serve Red Sangria (page 190), and for Easter, I make my colorful rainbow Sherbet Punch.

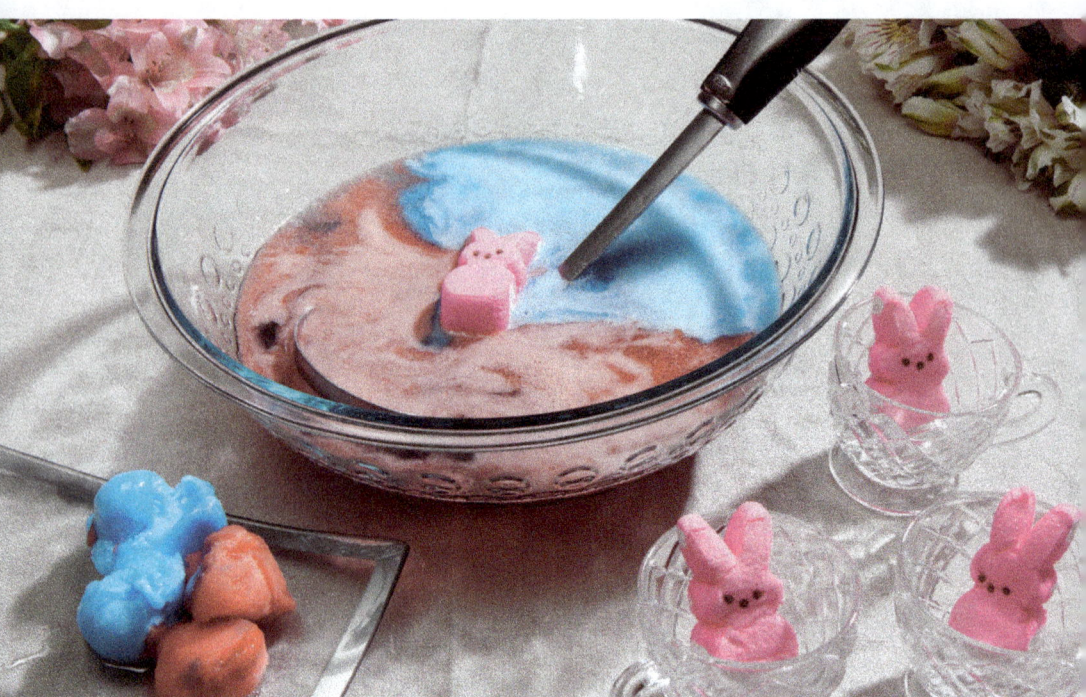

Sherbet Punch

2 (6-fluid-ounce) containers of Italian ice, any flavor
1 bottle rosé wine
1 cup ice cubes
¼ cup assorted colored marshmallows

Fill a punch bowl with ice. Add wine and Italian ice and combine. Top with a few marshmallows or Peeps.

If you are Italian and Catholic, then you can relate to being a child and sitting through midnight mass at Christmas or Easter. It is a three-hour event with every Catholic ceremony rolled up into one—baptisms, confirmations, you name it. It's incredibly beautiful, but as a child, it was challenging to sit still, especially being so full of Christmas excitement. However, it's quite a different experience going to the Easter vigil as a fifty-plus mom/wife than as a child. Although it is just as enjoyable, the feeling of wax dripping on my hand from the candle the last time I went caused me a little more heat than it would have when I was younger (when I was hot flash–free)! Yet humor helps us survive times like this. My husband looked over at me and wondered why I wasn't wearing my coat and said, "I thought you were cold." You are not supposed to laugh in church, but I'm pretty sure God forgives me that one.

Now that you have some party planning tips, get started! There's always an event to be celebrated. Maybe it's a friend getting a new job, you moving into a new place, or your son getting his first A in college. Find reasons to throw a party. In doing so, you will keep life light and fun. Laughter and celebrations are part of living our best lives in our fifties. In the next chapter, we will talk about how to break out of stale patterns and start living the life that you want. While it's not always comfortable, I'll encourage you to step out of the boundaries of the everyday and spice up and jazz up not just your meals but your entire life.

LUNGE POSE

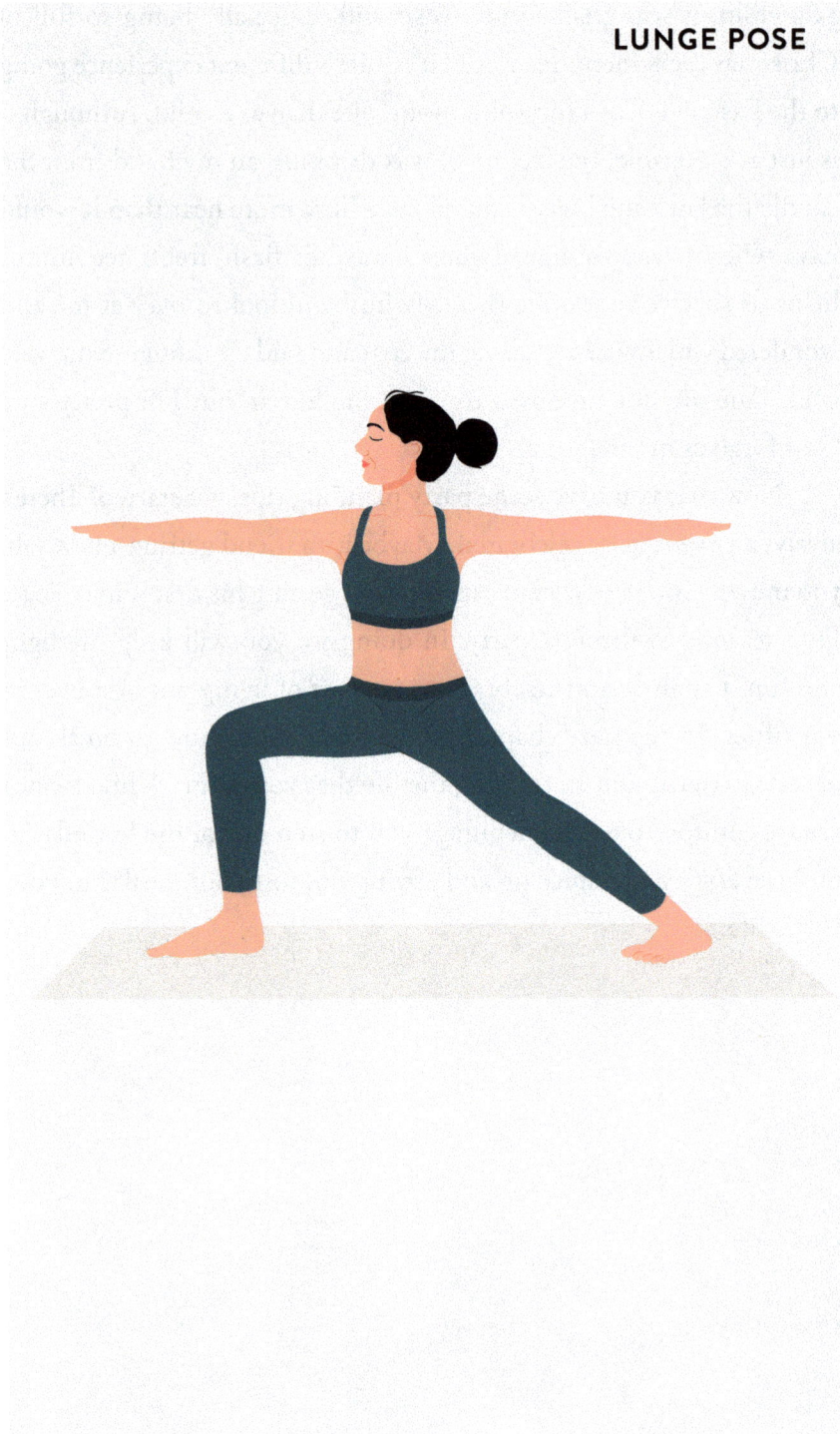

MOVE WITH MEANING

You've had a good workout doing chair squats; now it's time to stretch out your thighs with the yoga lunge pose. I consider this a working stretch. It isn't an easy position to hold, but it stretches your waist, ankles, knees, and legs. It also lengthens your spine and stimulates your gut to keep its contents moving (goodbye, bloat!). You can do this lunge with one knee on the floor, called a low lunge, but I like to do what is called a high lunge. Here's how:

1. Start in a standing position. With your hands on your hips, step your right foot forward about three feet. Keep your knee at a ninety-degree angle.
2. Distribute your weight evenly on both legs with your hips forward and square. Lift your left heel, pressing into the ball of your foot.
3. When you are steady, lift your arms high in the air, parallel to each other. Relax your shoulders.
4. Take ten deep breaths, then switch legs and repeat.

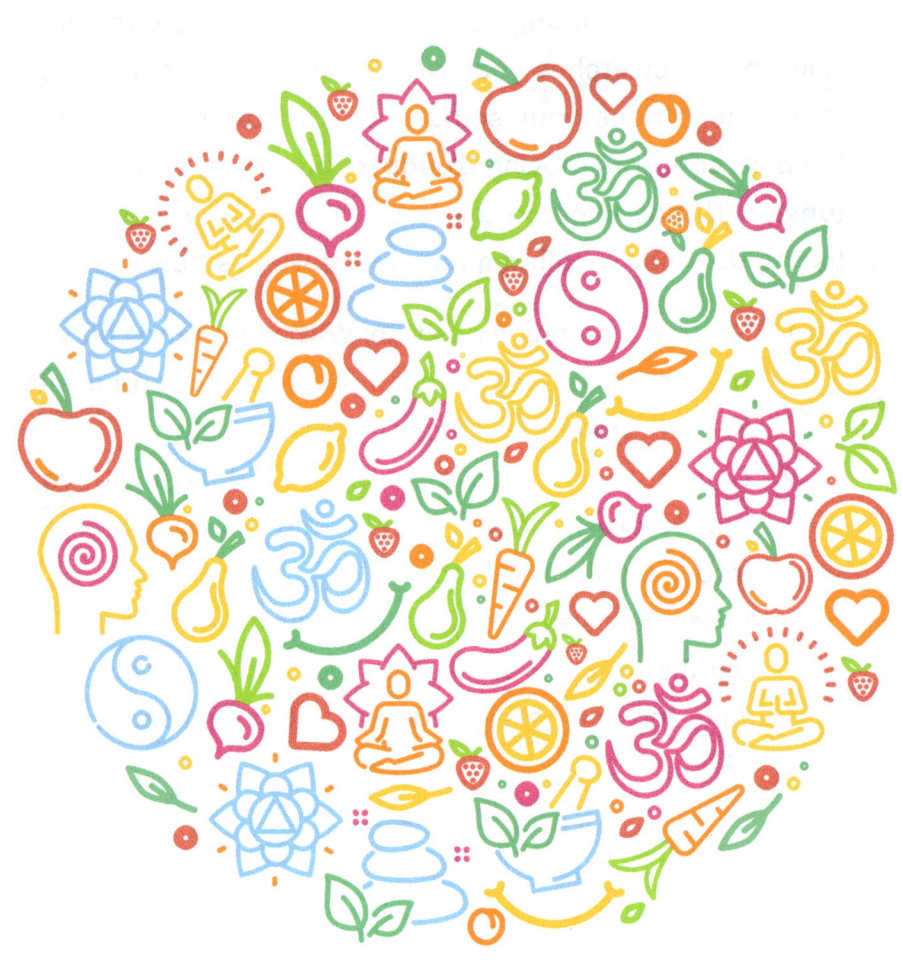

CHAPTER 12

Spice It Up, Jazz It Up
Sing a New Tune with Ceviche

Ever notice that when you do something on a whim that's out of the ordinary, it usually turns out to be incredibly fun or rewarding? My family owns a beach house on the Jersey Shore, and one day it was blistering hot at nearly 100°F. I didn't feel like jumping in the ocean, but I needed to cool off. I had to run to the store for supplies, and when I was there, I saw a baby pool. I thought, "That's the solution!" I bought two and brought them home and sat on the deck blowing them up. My family said, "Oh, that's so cute! You are going to put the dogs in them so they can cool off!" Nope. The pools were for me and whoever wanted to join me! I felt a little silly, but that just energized me to keep going. No one wanted to challenge me and tell me I was acting like a crazy lady. I made myself a signature drink, a White Sangria Spritzer with grapes (see chapter 8 for the recipe), and settled down into one of the pools. I felt like a million bucks! As I sat there, I thought, "I don't fear anyone but God."

Isn't it wonderful how growing older frees us from worrying about other people's opinions of us? It lets us act on impulses to do what we want to do without considering whether or not we are going to look silly or be ridiculed. As women, when we age we become like solid, sturdy little Buddhas. We hold this incredible calm and wisdom. We just have to listen and let it guide us. We are too smart, and we've lived too long and seen too much to do something really stupid. Add in that we don't care as much about other people's perceptions, and we are set free to jazz up and spice up our lives doing things that bring us pleasure and satisfaction. This gift is one of the very best things about being a woman in her fifties.

> **Your dreams won't come to you. You have to go to your dreams.**

I was never one to care too much about whether or not I looked silly, but I have noticed a healthy shift toward caring more about how I feel and checking in with myself about my own inner motivations and needs than about what others might think about my actions. I say follow your urges while applying your wisdom and take some risks and put yourself out there—even if it's as simple as sitting in a kiddie pool in your front yard! Or do something less daring, like making an out-of-the-ordinary dish like my husband's traditional Ecuadorean Ceviche.

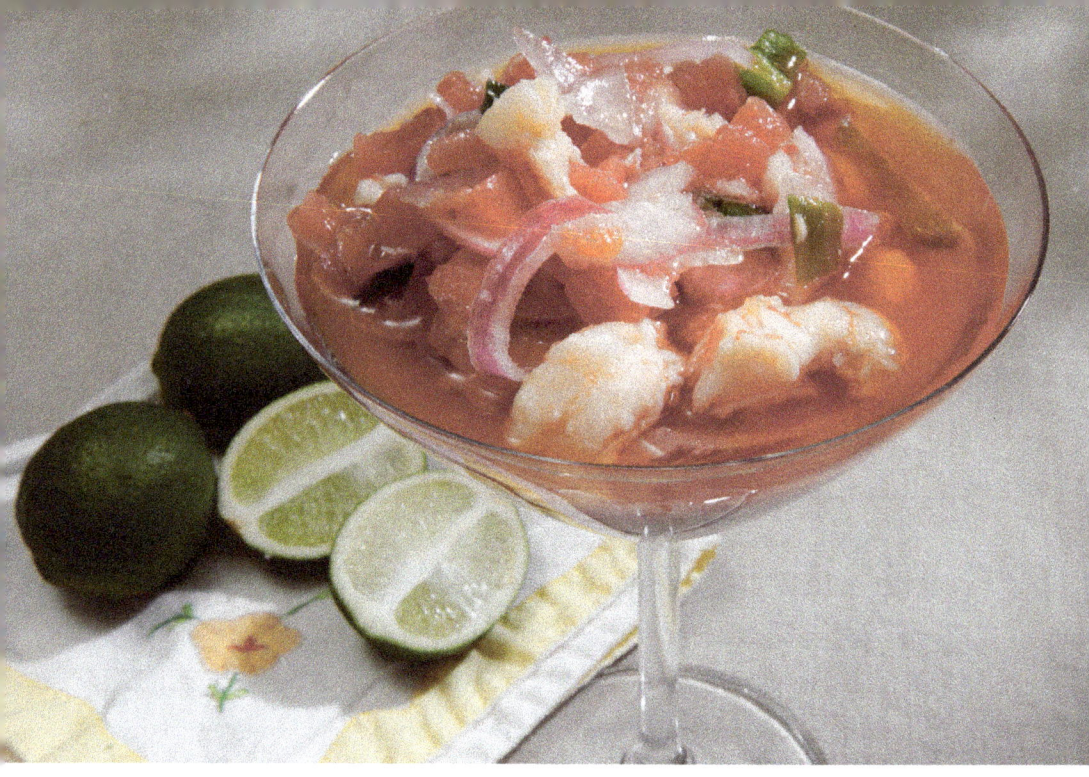

Ecuadorean Ceviche

- 1 small bag of limes
- 3 pounds shrimp
- 1 cup red onions
- ¼ cup salt
- ½ cup olive oil
- 3 scallions
- 1 green pepper
- 1 cup diced tomatoes

Clean and devein the shrimp and slice them in half. Lightly steam the shrimp. Finely chop the scallions and the green pepper. Slice the onion and dice the tomatoes. Mix shrimp and vegetables in a bowl with olive oil. Squeeze in juice from the limes, add salt, and combine well.

Being daring and stepping out of your comfort zone also applies to cooking. It's easy to get stuck in a rut with cooking. You go to the grocery store on autopilot and pick out the same food every week. That leads to eating the same meals day in and day out. Break out of the rut! And especially break out of salad hell. It's easy to think of salads as just simple greens, but there is so much more to do with salads. Spice them up! It's as simple as adding a few shakes of Tabasco or sriracha or sprinkling on pepper flakes and oregano. You can add spices to your salad or add them to your usual salad dressing for a zesty twist. Or dress up your green salad by switching out your greens. How about replacing iceberg lettuce with arugula, a spring mix, romaine, watercress, or even dandelion? My grandmother used to pick dandelions from the yard, put them in olive oil, and serve them up! Now that's living off the land.

Or try adding other favorite foods to your green salad. Think themes, like Italian, and add pepperoni or salami with a sprinkle of provolone cheese and some jarred roasted peppers. Yum! Or go Asian by adding edamame, tuna, sesame oil, and a dash of wasabi. Adding spice gives meals a zing and makes them absolutely electric. Salads are incredibly diverse and can become a meal with added protein. I try to eat a salad every day because they are so healthy. Being adventurous with your food is a great way to start jazzing up and spicing up your life by trying something out of your comfort zone. Start by making my Spicy Corkscrew Pasta Salad, with chili pepper.

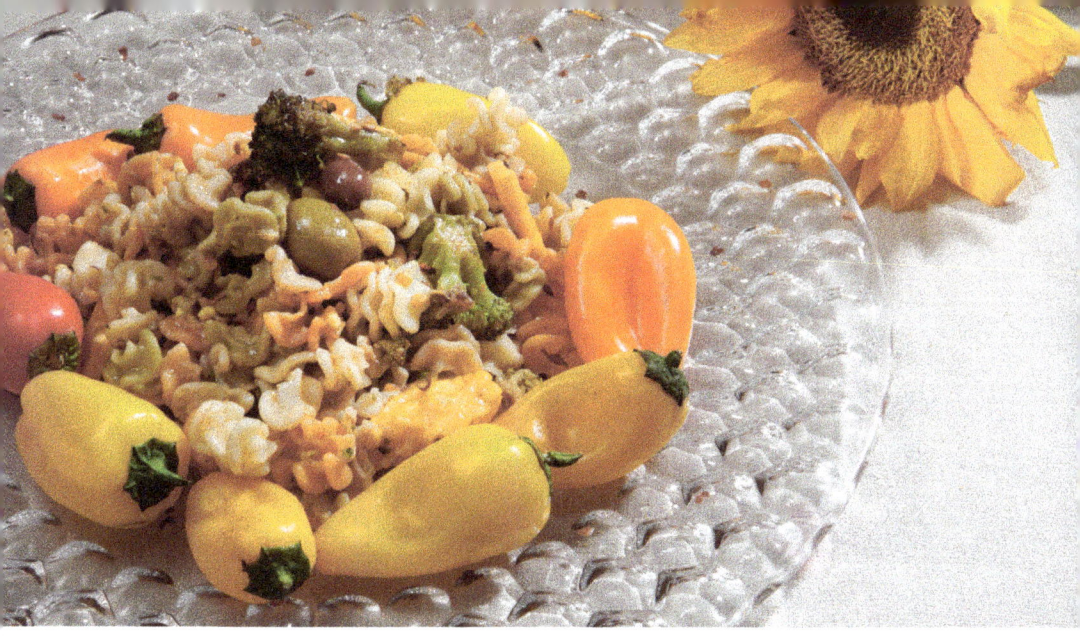

Spicy Corkscrew Pasta Salad

- 2 teaspoons chili pepper flakes
- ¼ cup bottled Italian dressing
- ¼ cup green and black olives
- 1 hard-boiled egg
- ¾ cup broccoli
- ½ avocado, sliced
- 2 teaspoons olive oil
- 1 garlic clove
- Dash salt
- ½ pound corkscrew pasta
- 1 cup cheddar cheese

Chop the green and black olives and slice the egg, avocado, and garlic. Cube the cheese. Boil and sauté the broccoli slightly in a pan with the olive oil, garlic, and salt. Prepare the pasta per directions. Combine all ingredients in a large bowl and enjoy.

You don't have to go so spicy that you need to douse your mouth with a fire extinguisher! I've eaten such spicy food that I could feel it burning my esophagus. One time my uncle ate a hot pepper in a restaurant, and he felt so desperate for relief that he grabbed the waiter and choked out the words, "Please get me water!" Even water couldn't cool him down. Another time, my brother-in-law mistook wasabi for guacamole and took a big bite. What a moment that was!

We all have a different level of comfort with spicy food and spicy living. My husband, Otto, has a big threshold for spicy. He can eat a whole plate of extra-hot food and he's just fine. I take one bite, and I go up to the ceiling like a ball of fire. Just like with life, you don't want to sprinkle on too much spice and take such a huge risk that you have a bad experience or put yourself in danger. On the other hand, you don't want to live such a bland life that everything becomes mundane and boring. Walk the middle line between adventure and comfort, and spicy food and bland.

Decide what is a little outside your comfort zone and give it a try. Traveling is a great opportunity to get your feet wet when it comes to taking risks. Traveling and vacation are inherently linked to adventure. When my kids were young, we took them to Ecuador to see where my husband grew up and to meet his family. We were totally spontaneous, which is not the way I usually roll, but I let go of the reins and let my husband lead. At one point, we were riding around in the back of a pickup truck with our two children. During the trip a praying mantis landed on Elissa's, my older daughter's, shirt. She had issues with insects, so she had quite the fright! I wanted my girls to experience unfiltered fun, and I knew we could keep them safe. I think they are better for it.

During that trip we would decide where to stay on the fly. If you haven't done that recently, give it a try! If you have older teenagers or kids in their early twenties, you probably watch them do it. They make weekend plans without really mapping things out, but in that impulsiveness blooms a ton of fun. How about planning a weekend away in a nearby town without making a hotel or dinner reservations, just winging it as you go along? See what happens. You might just have the adventure of your life.

Aging brings it home that we can't say to ourselves, "Someday I would like to do such-and-such." Someday is here! If there is something you have always wanted to do—whether it is skydiving, bungee jumping, writing a book of poems, or simply visiting somewhere special—do it! Now is the time. If you think you are too old, challenge yourself and do it. We have to live our lives to the fullest now while we plan for our futures, while we feel healthy and young. In our fifties, we are not retired yet, so we don't want to rest on our laurels. Whatever you put on hold to raise your kids, get back to it. There will only be more hurdles as we age.

A part of preventing those hurdles is obviously staying healthy physically with regular exercise and eating well. As we age, our bodies can quickly change, or an old injury can become chronic, causing us to give up our exercise routine. If that is happening to you, do something about it today. Call your doctor for an appointment or get a referral to a physical therapist. A friend of mine told me that her doctor said, "As you age, physical therapy is just something you will have to do now and then." Don't let physical setbacks stop you. Find solutions and keep moving. The better you can move, the more adventuring you can do.

> **Grow, don't shrink! You are no longer that insecure person. You left that person behind years ago.**

Life is simply sweeter (and spicier!) when we honor ourselves. When my mother-in-law passed away, I got a tattoo. I never thought in a million years that I would get a tattoo, but I did. It's a small cross with a heart that's on my shoulder, and it signifies Christ and love. It reminds me that religion is at the heart of me. When she died, it led me to realize that we all get just one life. It was my birthday shortly after, and that's when I got the tattoo, as a gift to myself. Maybe I was confronting my own mortality, but it makes me feel protected and reminds me to live life to the fullest.

Stepping out of your comfort zone is thrilling. Take a chance and do something new. It's magical. Tap into your childhood self and remember what it was like to be a child. Children don't always think; they act. They don't always see roadblocks or understand consequences; they just do what feels right. Get back to some of that hopeful, youthful joy and act. Even if it is doing something small, like mixing up your usual workout routine by getting outside and going on a hike or running on the beach instead of going to the gym, do it. When you take a risk or achieve a goal, pat yourself on your back and say, "I did it!"

Life is not a dress rehearsal. Stepping out of my comfort zone came to me as a habit later in life. Now I use Monday mornings to evaluate how I could make the week more exciting. Make a list and go for it. Use your imagination and wit because you've got it.

Don't be a chicken. I don't mean that in a cruel way. I have spent much of my life playing it safe, so it's advice to myself just as much as it's advice to you. Now I know that it's better to mess up and fail than to not try at all. When I stumble or start backing out, sometimes I stop and take a few deep yoga breaths and say three words to myself: "Take a step." I muster my confidence and take that next right step, and before I know it another follows. Have grit! You'll need it to face that little voice that throws out excuses or insults. Squash it and keep moving forward. Your best self is within you, ready to fly.

Challenge all those internal messages about what you can and can't do. What is a belief that you have about yourself that holds you back? Maybe it's that you are not athletic or not musical. Now, do something to prove that belief wrong. Join a sports team or take lessons, learn to play the piano, or whatever else appeals to you. Challenging those beliefs that make you say "I can't" helps you redefine yourself and see yourself in a new light. It opens the door to living a full and spicy life.

Sometimes when you are stepping out, it helps to have a partner in crime. It's okay to ask for support when trying something new. My sister-in-law came with me to get my tattoo, and I almost lost my nerve. It felt like a risk, but a safe one. Today, I get a little zing every time I look at it. It spices up my life! Just like my Sausage and Peppers will spice up yours.

Sausage and Peppers

> 1 pound hot sausage, sliced into thirds
>
> 2 bell peppers, sliced
>
> 2 tablespoons olive oil
>
> 1 jar tomato sauce
>
> ½ pound pasta

Sauté sausage and pepper slices in a frying pan with oil until sausage is cooked thoroughly. Add sauce. Transfer to cast-iron skillet and bake for 2 minutes at 350°F. Pour over prepared pasta and serve.

You've come a long way in life. You've made mistakes, you've seen things, and you have survived and grown. Instead of letting all that wisdom simply die with you, go out and put it to use. Jazz up and spice up your life. Every day, there's an opportunity to try something new or step outside your comfort zone. It's reassuring to have things set in life at this age, financially and with our relationships and careers, but it is also easy to sink into those comforts and forget to move. Instead, use your solid base as a launchpad to jump into a new way of being.

In our final chapter, things come full circle. We know how to live our best lives when it comes to eating well, exercising, and creating a life with meaning and joy. Relish in it! Join me in celebrating you in all your newfound glory and wisdom.

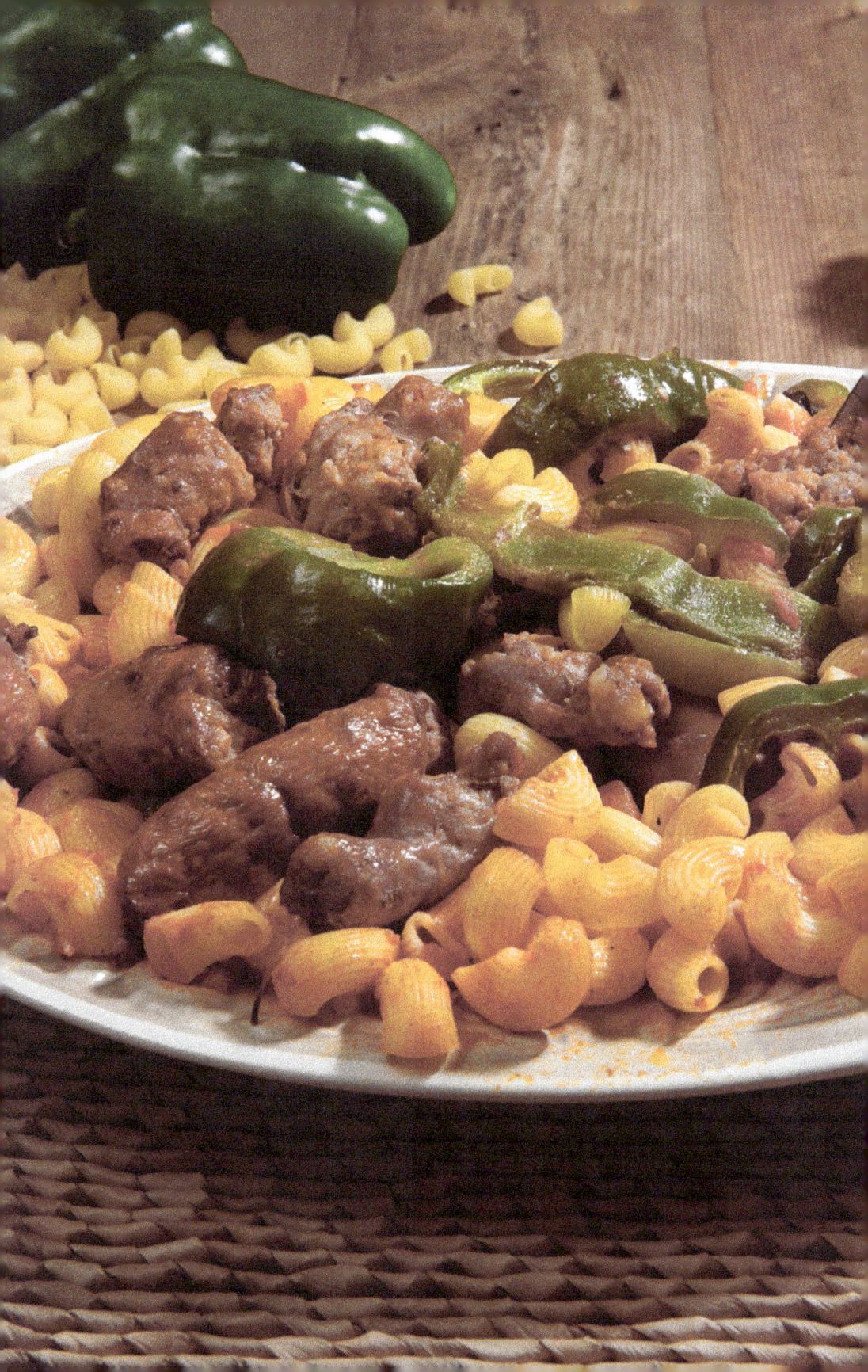

LOVING LIFE AT 50+

COBRA POSE

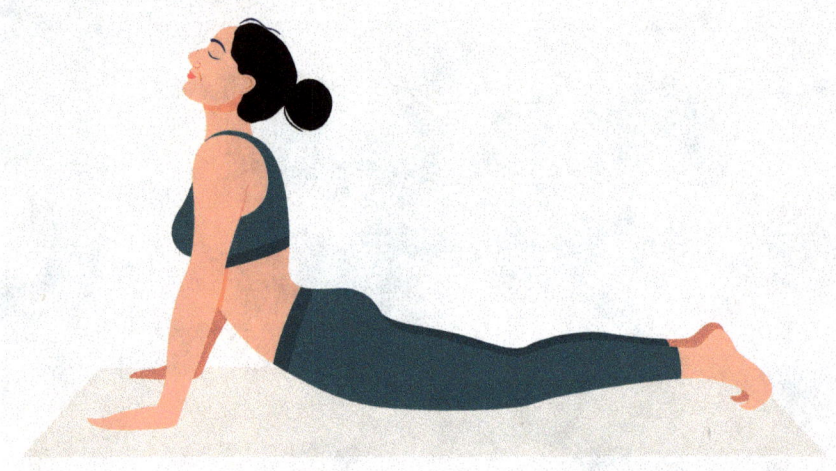

MOVE WITH MEANING

You've given your body a nice stretch with the yoga lunge position; now it's time to jazz it up with cobra pose. If you do it right, it will feel a little uncomfortable, like the back bends you used to do as a kid in gym class, but it warms and opens your chest. You are doing a cobra with lift versus a cobra where you remain on the floor. In yoga tradition, cobra pose signifies your ability to overcome your fear and to find your power. Dive in:

1. Drop down to your knees. Rest on your palms, which are flat and aligned with your shoulders.
2. Stretch your legs out behind you and lie down on the floor. Hug your elbows to your sides and keep your legs and pelvis steady and solid. Take a calming breath.
3. When you feel steady, inhale and lift your chest and body off of the floor. Keep your gaze level and neck neutral.
4. Hold the pose and your breath for ten to fifteen seconds. Then exhale and drop to the floor. Repeat five times.

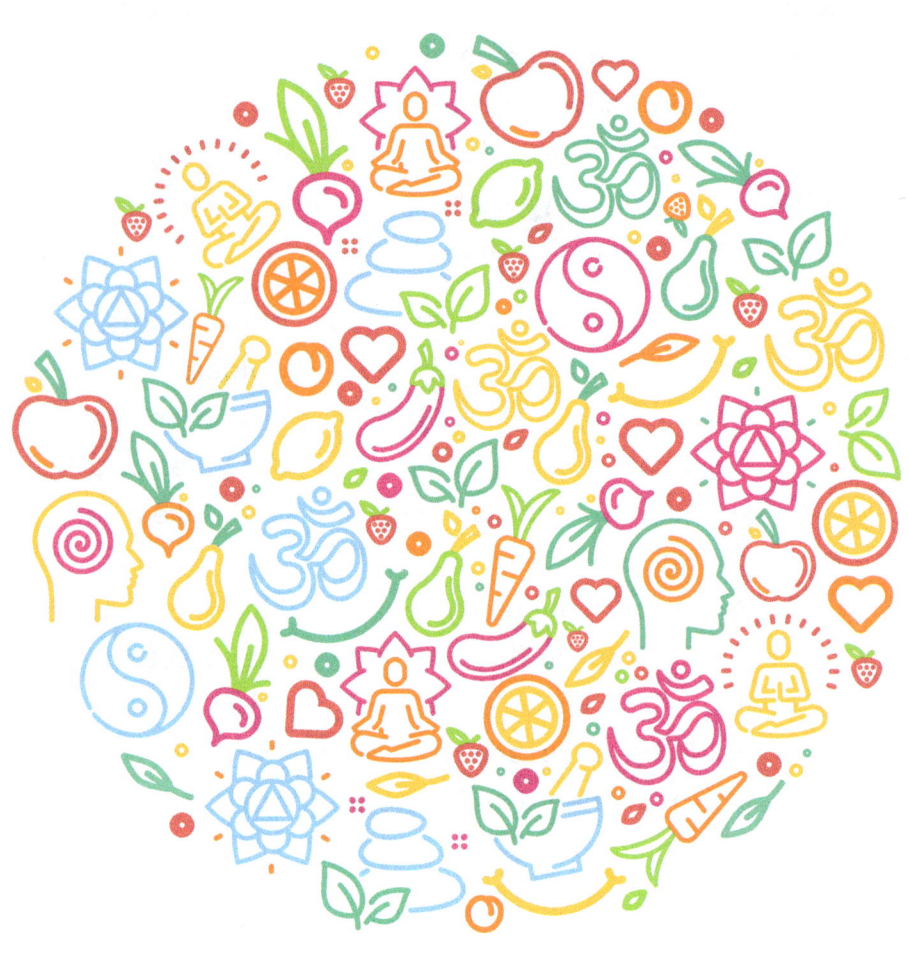

CHAPTER 13

Feast on Life
Feel Satisfied with a Surprising Brown Rice Salad

I recently took a trip to Italy with my family. It wasn't my first time visiting, but this time I wanted to focus on sharing good food and adventures together. My girls are young and in that late-teen/early-twenties invincible stage when you feel like anything is possible. One day, they pushed me way outside my comfort zone, helping me practice what I preach! We signed up for a boat trip to see caverns and hidden beaches around Sorrento, in the Gulf of Naples. I had to take two motion sickness pills just to get on the small boat, but I am so glad that I did. The sights we saw were breathtaking. It felt like we were on the edge of the earth! It was a shock to our senses, waking us up to the beauty and wonders of our wild blue planet.

At the end of the boat trip, we could either take an elevator up the cliff and then hail a taxi to our hotel, or we could hike. In the spirit of our adventure, we decided to hike up the cliff and walk to our hotel instead. It felt like I was in boot camp. By the time we made it to the top, I felt amazing. I was sweaty and hot but totally pumped. Going fast on a boat, then accomplishing a hike I didn't think was possible was extremely gratifying.

By now you have fully grasped my three-pronged approach to living your best life in your fifties: (1) eating well, (2) exercising and enjoying it, and (3) being mindful to bring experiences and people into your life that fulfill you and bring you joy. When you have this winning trifecta in motion on a regular basis, you can't help but feel satisfied and happy with your life. Your worries about the future and growing older drop away because you are loving life *today*. You are awake and aware and present in every moment, soaking in life and acting intentionally to create the life you want.

Being in Italy satisfied all three of these elements of a contented life. We ate healthy, fresh food, we exercised simply by walking, swimming, and taking in the views, and we reveled in one another's company as we enjoyed our adventures. Think of it as a three-pronged wheel that when continually spinning propels you into your best self and your best life.

I checked my dream of sharing delicious food in Italy with my family off my Big Dream Bucket List from chapter 6. It was almost like tasting food for the first time. Enjoying it with my family, the people I love the most in the world, made it all the more delicious. Truly, it affirmed for me why God made food!

Italians make every meal an event. Every meal had pearls of ecstasy: olive oil so freshly pressed that I was tempted to bathe in it, thick wedges of parmigiana cheese, freshly twisted mozzarella, and vine-ripened vegetables like tomato, eggplant, and zucchini. My favorite dishes were *frutti di mare* (fresh fruit of the sea—i.e., seafood) and other seafood dishes, like mussel linguini and rich clam sauces.

In Italy, all meals end with scrumptious desserts of fresh fruits, figs, or gelato followed by sips of limoncello and the last swallows of succulent red wines. Don't forget about the cappuccino and espresso, born in Italy and like nowhere else on earth. It was like tasting the beauty of the landscape around us, the majestic mountains and the striking blue sea.

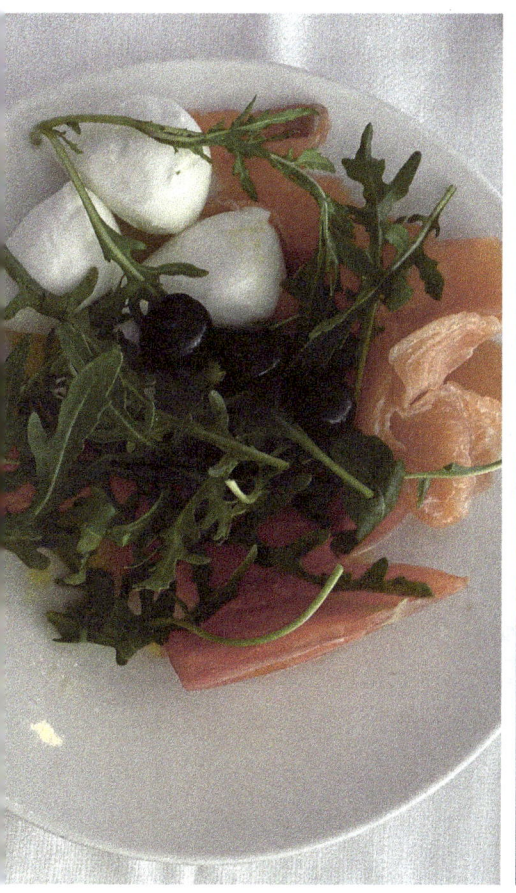 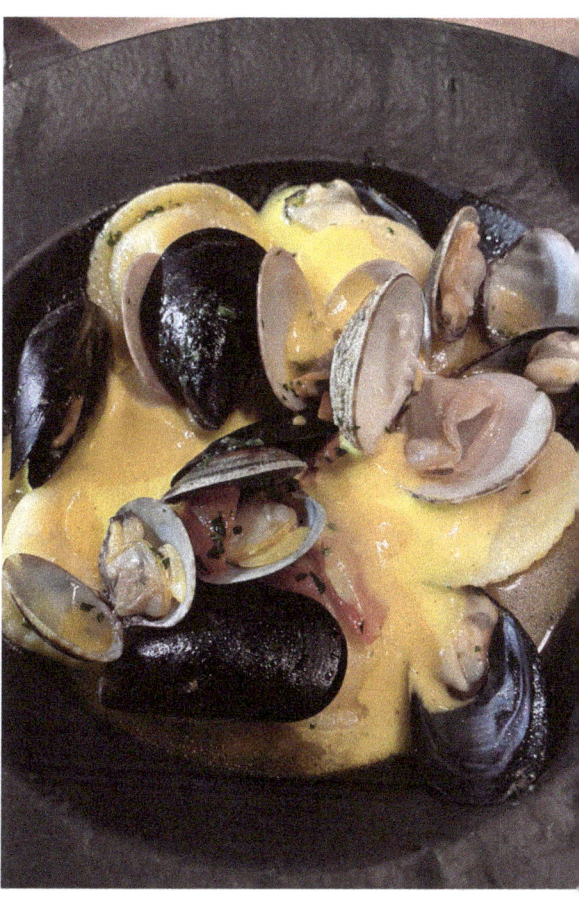

(L) Simple Italian seafood salad with fresh fish, mozzarella, olives and arugula. Look at that presentation! (R) Fresh olive oil added an incredible richness to this Italian mussel sauce.

Before leaving for Italy, I went to the WNDR Museum in Chicago with my youngest daughter, Emily. There was a booth where you could write down a saying that defines your life. The words "All you need is love" immediately came to mind. I know they are familiar Beatles lyrics, but they are profound in their simplicity. Love is at the root of who we are and where we come from. Love is family. And part of loving your family is loving yourself. Knowing what brings us meaning and satisfaction in the present lets us move forward and live our best lives in the future. So go for it. If you want to write that book, open that boutique, or go on a cruise down the Danube, it's time. Take that leap of faith. No matter what, don't sleep through your life or sit in the passenger seat. Be the driver!

Remember, people who are the most successful are not the smartest; they just work the hardest. And they have confidence, even when they are afraid. Writing this book and sharing my recipes was way out of my comfort zone. When I was preparing the food for the photographs featured in the book, I made every recipe within two weeks. The photographer was so meticulous. Everything had to be just right. I wasn't sure I could do it, but all of a sudden I shifted into gear, and my inner pastry chef and line cook came out, and I got it just right! I couldn't believe I had it in me, and to know it was there all along was such a confidence boost.

Before deciding to write this book, I watched *Chopped* and other cooking shows every night, and I felt so inspired. Cooking and learning about food feeds my brain. With my career, I need to both feed my intellect and satisfy my psyche. Financial gain is not the focus. It means the world to share myself with you. It helps me feel connected. We are not alone; we have a support network of beautiful, interesting women in their fifties and beyond. Tap into your community and give each other wings to fly. Grow every day; if not for yourself, then do it for the ones you love.

Opportunity is knocking all the time. Decide to listen and open the door.

Stay hungry! Not literally, I don't want you to starve. I simply want you to stay focused and aware as you go through your days. Be conscious of what you put in your mouth and savor every bite. Don't eat standing up or in a rush. Sit; chew; enjoy. When you make good food that's healthy, you feel satiated in more ways than one. Stay mindful of the food that you buy and the meals you prepare, and avoid setting yourself up for eating too little and wanting to make up for it later with mindless munching.

Practice my simple, proven habits for maintaining a healthy weight through healthy eating in chapter 4, which include watching your portion size, never skipping meals, eating on a schedule, being aware of calories, and not letting the scale rule you. When you step on a scale, weigh it all, including how much you are exercising, how much you are enjoying every moment with your friends and family, and especially everything that you are grateful for in life. Weight is not just a number on a scale; it's about how you feel and how you move. It's about feeling filled up by things other than food and keeping the idea that eating well is inherently linked to feeling well and being happy. Remember that eating healthy is not simply about looking good; it's really about feeling your best and knowing you are doing the right thing for your body, like eating my tasty Brown Rice Salad. It's my favorite healthy vegetarian recipe, hands down.

LOVING LIFE AT 50+

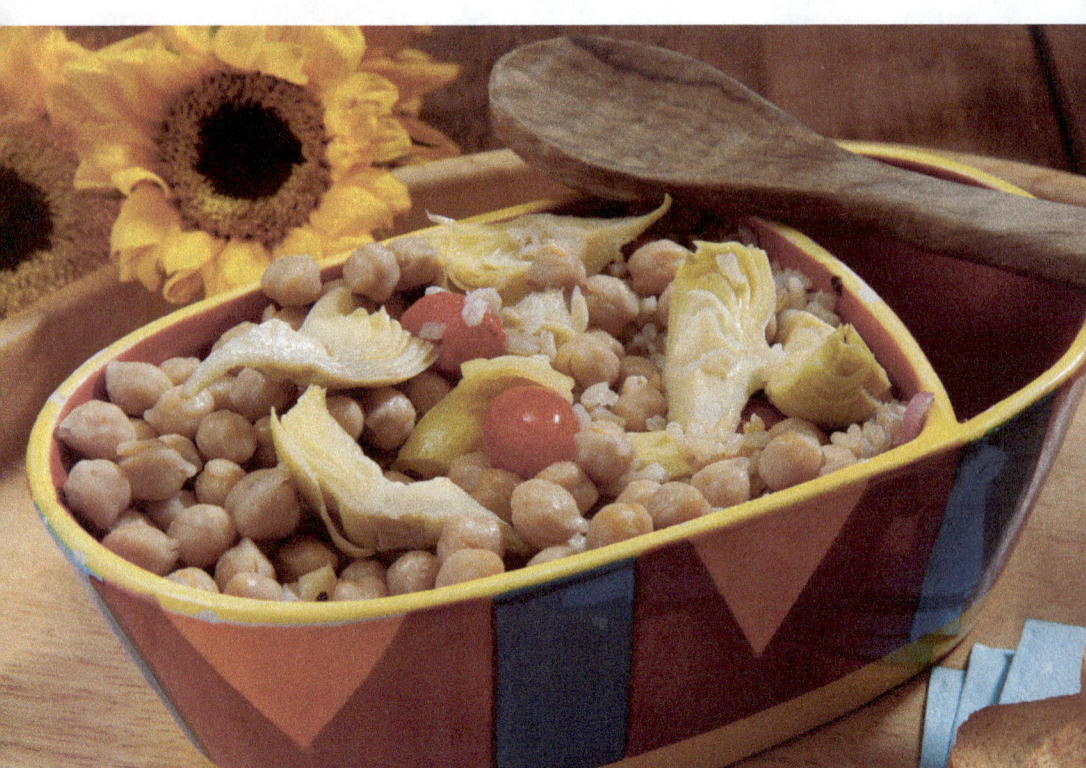

Brown Rice Salad

- 10 ounces brown rice, cooked
- 4 ounces marinated jarred artichokes, drained
- 1 (14-ounce) can garbanzo beans, drained
- 1 teaspoon oregano
- 1 teaspoon salt
- 1 cup cherry tomatoes, halved
- ¼ cup chopped red onion
- 1 can drained tuna (optional)
- 2 teaspoons olive oil

Combine all ingredients. Serve cold.

The same goes for exercising every day and finding activities that are fun that you naturally want to do. Find your personal yoga (maybe it's yoga!). Once you find it, do it every day. If you need more inspiration for getting active, revisit chapter 2. A hard workout is extremely affirming, like when I climbed what felt like a mountain in Sorrento. Keep a youthful mentality as you age and never lose your sense of humor.

Remember, you can practice all three healthy habits at one time by turning your kitchen into a dance studio and dancing like a diva as you prepare a delicious meal to share with friends or family—meals like my juicy Skillet Chicken Thighs. They are the perfect main course for a family dinner.

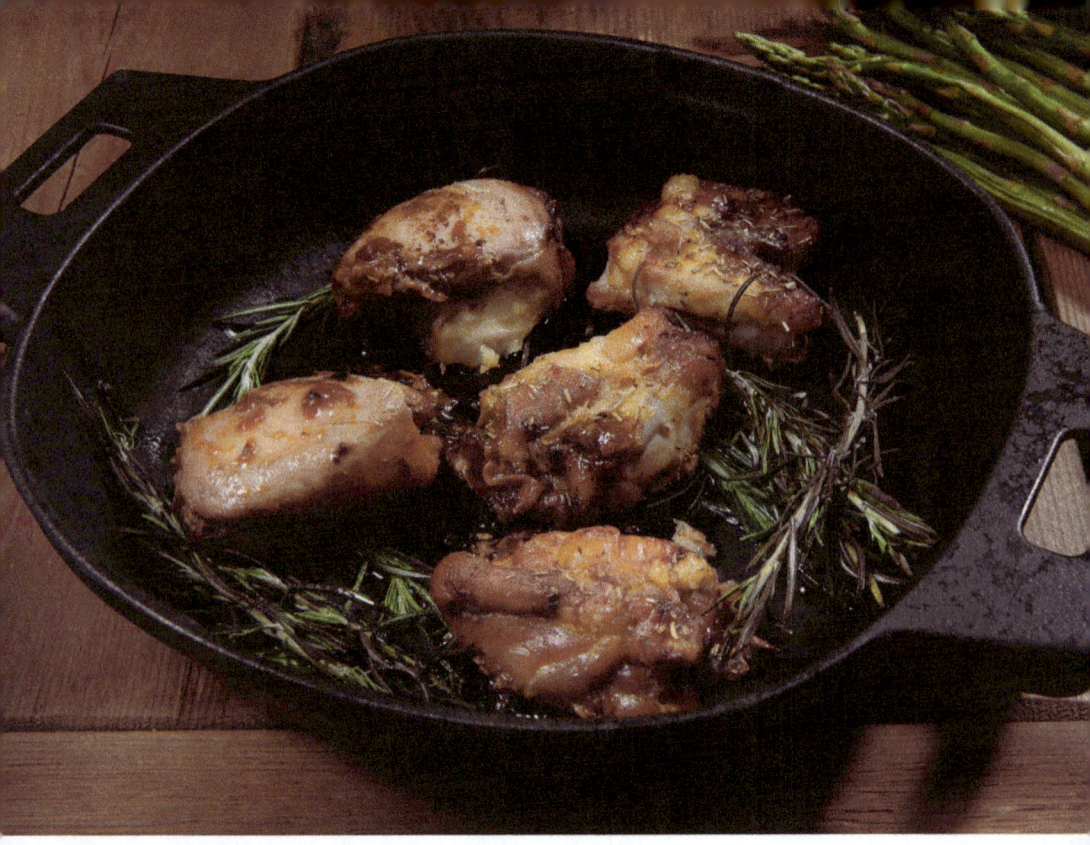

Skillet Chicken Thighs

2 pounds chicken thighs, marinated*
3 teaspoons olive oil
Salt and pepper, to taste

For marinade:
¼ cup red wine
3 teaspoons balsamic glaze

Make marinade and rub on chicken, letting it sit for 30 minutes in the refrigerator. Panfry marinated thighs in warm oil. Add salt and pepper. Cook thoroughly for about 30 minutes, turning over several times to brown both sides. If preferred, bake in oven for 25 minutes at 375°F.

Challenge yourself physically. Did you always want to do a marathon but now that feels way out of reach? Sign up for a 5K. Do you want to learn a new sport or exercise technique? Enroll in a class through your gym or your city's recreation center. Pick the class that sounds f-u-n, like Zumba, dance, tennis, or yoga in the park. Even when you feel tired after work, do something. It can be less than you planned when you felt motivated in the morning. Plans change. Then pat yourself on the back for getting up and moving. There's simply no room for self-judgment these days!

You've arrived. Look forward to the future and enjoy your fifties with no regrets. Do what makes you happy. You are a diva! An awesome woman who can rise above in this world of ups and downs. Go live your life. It's a crazy, wonderful world, and you were blessed to be born into it, so make the most of your one, authentic life. Feast on all the flavors, whether it's food, friends, family, or active fun. Jump in and step out dripping with joy, self-appreciation, and love. I'm right here with you. I promise.

SAVASANA POSE

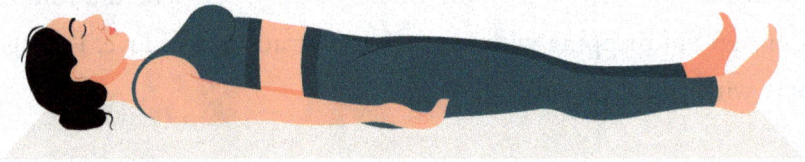

MOVE WITH MEANING

Every good yoga practice has a cooldown routine. Part of the cooldown routine is a Savasana pose. This pose is deeply satisfying. You are relaxed and awakened to future possibilities. As you relax, with your arms by your side, release any negative thoughts that are weighing you down. It is tempting to fall asleep in this position, but it is a time for taking stock, reveling in life, and relaxation. Doesn't that sound familiar? In your fifties, you don't want to sleepwalk through life; you want to stay alert to possibilities while maintaining a good balance between health and pleasure.

Thank you for taking this journey with me. Fifty is not the new forty or the new sixty, but it is the time to embrace life with humor and wellness.

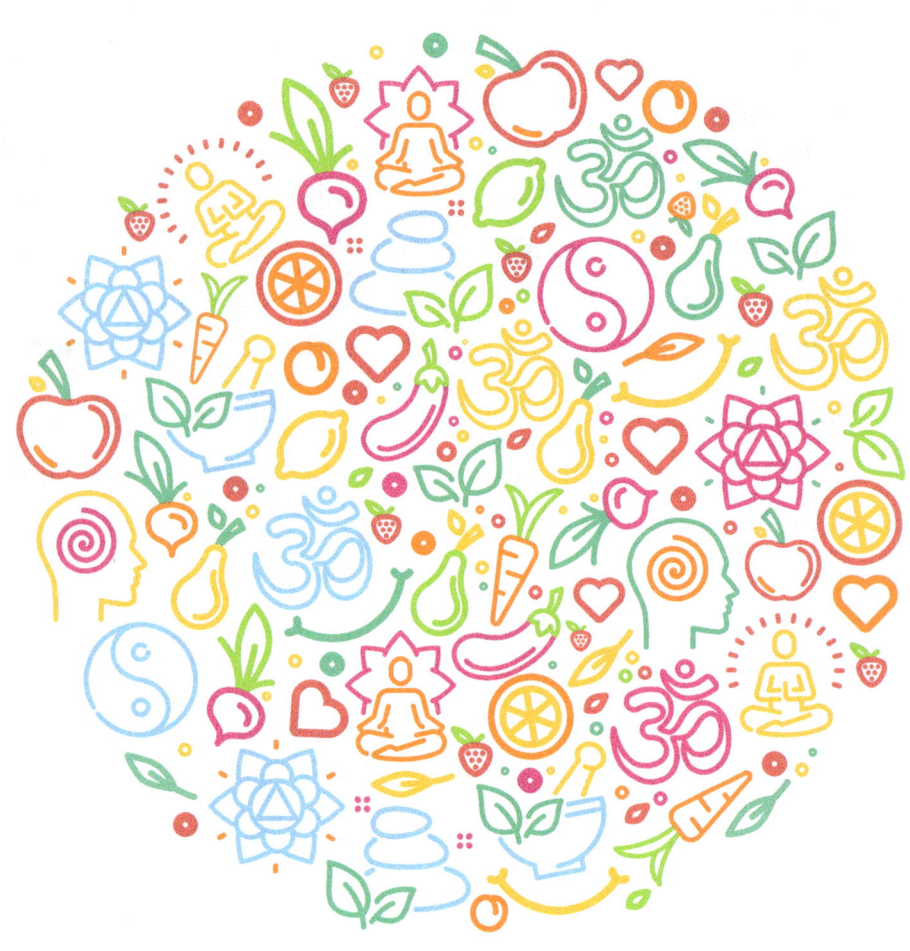

ABOUT THE AUTHOR

Maria Sabando is part chef, part yoga aficionado, and a little bit Italian diva. This Georgetown University grad puts her life experience of teaching yoga, selling makeup, cooking, and being a mother to good use. She's constantly simmering with new ideas for recipes, life hacks, and ways to squeeze the most out of life.

www.ingramcontent.com/pod-product-compliance
Lightning Source LLC
Chambersburg PA
CBHW050523170426
43201CB00013B/2063